200 best

L
ee
pes

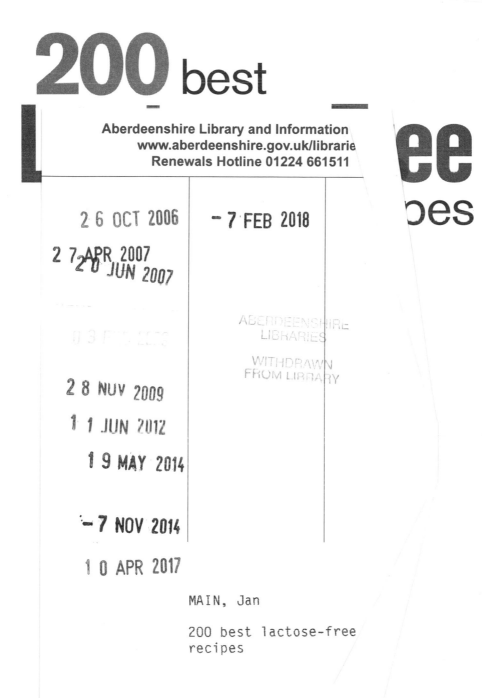

MAIN, Jan

200 best lactose-free
recipes

200 best
Lactose-Free
recipes

From appetizers and soups
to main courses and desserts

Jan Main

Robert
ROSE

For complete cataloguing information, see page 276.

Disclaimer
This is a cookbook and does not contain medical or dietary advice. Any questions regarding the impact of diet and health should be directed to your physician. The Publisher and the Author specifically disclaim any liability, loss or risk, personal or otherwise, which is incurred as a consequence, directly or indirectly, of the use and application of any of the contents of this book.

Design & Production: PageWave Graphics Inc.
Editor: Sue Sumeraj
Proofreader: Sheila Wawanash
Recipe Testers: Lesleigh Landry, Sandy Spurgeon, Lucy Gray and Jacqui Humphrey
Indexer: Gillian Watts
Photography: Colin Erricson (cover photo) and Mark T. Shapiro (backcover photos)
Food Stylist: Kate Bush
Props Stylist: Charlene Erricson

Cover image: Fudge Pudding (page 232)

We acknowledge the financial support of the Government of Canada through the Book Publishing Industry Development Program (BPIDP) for our publishing activities.

Published by: Robert Rose Inc.
120 Eglinton Ave. E., Suite 800, Toronto, Ontario, Canada M4P 1E2
Tel: (416) 322-6552 Fax: (416) 322-6936

Printed in Canada
1 2 3 4 5 6 7 8 9 10   CPL   15 14 13 12 11 10 09 08 07 06

To my food friends and to Rhoda,
whose enduring support spurred me on.

Contents

Preface 8

Acknowledgments 9

Introduction 10

Dips, Spreads and Other Nibbles 23

Breakfast, Brunch and Lunch 51

Soups 67

Salads 83

Pasta and Pizza 105

Main Courses 131

Side Dishes 159

Breads 175

Desserts 205

Sauces, Spreads and Toppings 241

Smoothies and Other Beverages 263

Appendix I: Celebration Menus 272

Appendix II: Nutrient Analysis 275

Index 277

Preface

For lactose-intolerant individuals, the experience of enjoying delicious meals without a tell-tale rumble from their tummy can be a rare event. They can't imagine sitting down to eat without having to have at least some special foods, as well as having to pass on tempting dishes reserved for others.

200 Best Lactose-Free Recipes ends this isolation. Jan Main has selected recipes that for years have been forbidden territory for many people with lactose intolerance. Cream soups, salmon mousse, béchamel sauce, rice pudding, cheesecake, tiramisu and ice creams are just a few of the delights that have been off-limits in the past.

This is not a textbook on living a lactose-free life. Instead, it is a beautifully written and well-presented guidebook to tasty, healthy food that lactose-intolerant people can enjoy. The topic has been carefully researched to find substitutions that not only eliminate or substantially reduce lactose levels, but also provide additional health benefits. The reader gets a chance to increase knowledge of the importance of calcium in the diet and learn what will and will not work to enhance the supply of that mineral to the body. Thus the introduction and use of tofu (prepared with calcium salts) to enhance the calcium content of a recipe. This is definitely a plus for lactose-intolerant people, since even though there are good dairy choices available, they are often rejected for fear of an adverse reaction.

The numerous tips and hints provided will benefit cooks of all abilities. The introduction provides useful information on tofu and soy milk — possibly new ingredients in a cook's repertoire. Lactose-free milk is also utilized, and is perhaps introduced to some for the first time.

200 Best Lactose-Free Recipes is a welcome addition to the kitchen libraries of people with lactose intolerance and others who enjoy tasty, interesting food.

Marsha Rosen, RD

Acknowledgments

A book is never written in isolation. There are a number of people whose help, enthusiasm and interest were a tremendous inspiration and kept me at it:

- my students, who first planted the seed of writing a cookbook
- Khristina Weinacht, lactose intolerant herself, who suggested the topic
- Janice Daciuk, whose dietetic background, love of baking and organizational skills made testing recipes a joy
- Marsha Rosen for her gracious support
- Lesleigh Landry, Sandy Spurgeon, Lucy Gray and Jacqui Humphrey for their testing competence
- my friends and family who critique the successes with the failures

There are many more thank yous to be said, but to those people I give a personal thank you so this may remain succinct.

Introduction

In this book you'll find recipes for all meals and every occasion, suitable for friends and family to enjoy regardless of their tolerance to milk. My goal was to produce lactose-free recipes that taste great!

Recipes included are of two types:

- those based on milk that have been revamped with lactose-free soy foods, lactose-free milk, fruit juice and stock
- those that make a significant contribution to calcium.

Many people ask me if I am lactose intolerant and hence my interest in this topic. No, I am not, at least not at this point, but I do have an array of inconvenient food allergies, which makes me sympathetic to the cause. My friend Christina, newly diagnosed with lactose intolerance, suggested I write this cookbook to help her. It made sense as I began to understand her predicament. Christina is a wonderful cook of Hungarian background. She loved making cream-filled tortes, creamy sauces and cheese dishes. You can imagine her frustration. Even a drop of milk in her cup of tea caused discomfort.

At this time, I was teaching a cooking class to a Chinese group, all lactose intolerant. They have been excellent teachers to me! At one of our first classes we did a kulebiaka of salmon, always popular with past classes. I observed with some concern and wonder as the women happily tucked into the asparagus salad, gobbled down the Atlantic salmon with the wild rice and mushroom stuffing, ate sparingly of the green mayonnaise, and only tasted the flaky, buttery pastry that enveloped the salmon. My first lesson. The rich foods with sour cream and butter caused this lactose-intolerant group digestive problems.

Tofu was my next lesson. This same group introduced me to their tofu, superior to the tofu of my experience from a supermarket vegetable counter. This tofu had a delicate flavor and texture; in fact, it reminded me of custard. They told me how to care for tofu and different ways to prepare it. All news to me. Five pounds of tofu can go a long way in recipe experimentation! When I discovered that, in addition to the creamy texture tofu gives dishes, it is also a calcium source if made with calcium chloride or calcium sulfate, I began to realize the potential for tofu in lactose-free cooking.

As I have researched and tested recipes for this book, I have learned to bake without butter, make delectable sauces without cream and use only a whiff of hard cheese for flavor. You do not need to feel deprived if you are lactose intolerant!

Lactose Intolerance Defined

Lactose is the milk sugar found in all animal milk, including human milk. Lactose intolerance is the inability to digest this milk sugar. Most of us are born with lactase, an enzyme found in the digestive tract, which breaks lactose down into two simple sugars: glucose and galactose. If lactase is no longer available to break down lactose into these two simple sugars, the sugar goes on to the large intestine, where it becomes fermented by intestinal bacteria. This fermentation causes the symptoms of lactose intolerance — bloating, diarrhea, abdominal pain and gas. Symptoms will vary from individual to individual. With prolonged diarrhea, there are the side effects of rectal tenderness, dehydration, weakness and weight loss. Some people will be uncomfortable while, on rare occasions, others will have to be hospitalized.

Primary Intolerance

When lactose intolerance occurs due to the decline in lactase, it is considered primary intolerance. Between the ages of five and seven the activity of this enzyme often declines, and many of the world's adults lose their ability to digest lactose. In fact, most of the world's population cannot digest milk — only Western and Northern Europeans tolerate milk. Many Asians, Hispanics, people from Mediterranean nations, Blacks and Native North Americans are lactose intolerant.

Secondary Intolerance

When lactose intolerance occurs as a result of a disease, this is classed as a secondary intolerance. Some diseases that might result in lactose intolerance are ulcerative colitis, celiac disease, Crohn's disease, viral diarrhea or cancer. In these cases, a reduced-lactose diet is recommended while the symptoms persist and until the system settles down. Once the enzyme begins to work again, regular dairy foods can be reintroduced. If enzyme depletion is permanent, milk containing lactose cannot be reintroduced. Fortunately, there are lactose-free milks available, as well as tablets that can be taken with milk foods to help digest the lactose. A doctor should be consulted for assistance, and a dietitian can help with an appropriate diet.

Milk Allergy

Milk allergy is quite different from lactose intolerance. It is a reaction to the protein in milk, not the sugar, and affects the immune system, causing classic allergy symptoms — wheezing, eczema, rash, mucus buildup, and asthma. Milk allergy usually affects babies or young children and can be serious. The child will be put on a soy formula because to continue with milk will only assault the immune system further. Often the child will outgrow the allergy. Once this happens, milk and milk products can gradually be reintroduced into the diet, but parents should check with the doctor to find out when and if milk can be reintroduced.

Diagnosing Lactose Intolerance

If you suspect you are lactose intolerant, have your condition checked by your doctor. The doctor may do one of several tests to determine if this is the problem.

Once you are diagnosed, your doctor or dietitian will put you on a lactose-free diet to clear your system. That means no milk and no products that contain milk, such as whey, curds, cheese, yogurt, sour cream, ice cream, sherbets, butter or margarine containing milk products or cottage cheese.

Each person is affected differently. You may experience discomfort from bloating and diarrhea, but still be able to function. Or you may be quite ill, and it will take longer to return to a healthy balance. You will be put on a plain diet, eating easily digested food such as steamed vegetables and fish with lots of clear fluids. You should get plenty of rest and cut out caffeine and alcohol. Once your system has calmed down, you can gradually reintroduce small amounts of food that contain lactose.

Finding Your Tolerance Level

As a lactose-intolerant patient, you will receive helpful information from your doctor or dietitian on how to find your tolerance to milk products. It is important to find your tolerance to milk and dairy products because of their nutrition contribution to your diet.

Every person has a different tolerance level. Some can have yogurt; some cannot. Some can tolerate hard natural cheese (as opposed to soft unripened cheese); some cannot. For some, milk or milk products eaten in small quantities with a meal are easier to digest. It is a trial and error method unique to each individual, and results vary with each individual from time to time.

Start with the most easily digested milk products first and work your way up to find your tolerance level. Remember to go slowly and wait a day before adding another food.

Foods in Order of Ease of Digestion for the Lactose Intolerant

1. Plain breads and baked goods
2. Fermented dairy foods such as yogurt, in which the live bacteria help you digest the lactose more easily.
3. Hard aged cheeses with low lactose levels such as aged Cheddar, Gouda, Edam and Parmesan.
4. If all goes well, try about ¼ cup (50 mL) of milk and work up to 1 cup (250 mL) over several days.

Tolerance will also vary according to the level of stress in your life. You may normally tolerate yogurt, but if a particular week is difficult, your symptoms may return. You will have to learn to judge.

It is reassuring to know that, for many lactose-intolerant people, the enzyme available in tablet form can help improve their tolerance levels. By taking two or more tablets before eating a food containing lactose, the symptoms are often eliminated or greatly reduced.

Obvious Sources of Lactose

Milk and milk products — chocolate milk, skim, whole and 1% milk, skim milk powder, goat's milk products, cottage cheese, ricotta cheese, whipping (35%) cream, half-and-half (10%) cream, light (5%) cream, yogurt, buttermilk, sour cream, ice cream, ice milk, sherbet, milk puddings.

Not-So-Obvious Sources of Lactose

Cereals produced with skim milk powder, processed meats such as sausages and wieners, commercially prepared creamed vegetable dishes such as scalloped potatoes or vegetables in a sauce, cream soups, commercial pancakes and waffles, cake mixes, muffin mixes, milk chocolate, chocolate drink mixes, certain prepared cakes, breads, pies and cookies, medications.

You need to know how to read ingredient listings on food labels to know if lactose is present in a particular food. Lactose is present when the label includes milk, milk solids, cheese flavor, whey, curds, or margarine, unless labeled "non-dairy." Lactose is not present when the ingredient listing includes lactic acid, lactalbumin, lactate, or casein. Ingredients are listed in order of the greatest quantity to the smallest; therefore, where the ingredient falls in the list will give you some idea of the relative amount in the food.

Small amounts of lactose are added during the processing of numerous foods and drug products. Check with your pharmacist in the case of medications.

The Importance of Milk and Milk Products
Vitamin D

Milk is fortified with Vitamin D, sometimes called the sun vitamin, which prevents us from getting rickets, a disease causing bone deformity and stunted growth. It is essential for the absorption of calcium. Vitamin D is only available in fortified milk, fortified soy milk, fish oils (cod liver oil and halibut oil) and from exposure to the sun. When the skin is exposed to the sun, it manufactures vitamin D. If you are unable to drink milk and have limited access to daily sun, or wear sun block, it may be a good idea to take a supplement, but check with your doctor or dietitian first to learn your individual needs. Too much vitamin D can be toxic.

Calcium

Milk and milk products are excellent sources of calcium. In fact, nutrition guidelines often recommend daily servings of milk and milk products from infancy to old age. Obviously, if you are lactose intolerant, you may not be able to consume the recommended quantity of milk.

Fortunately, milk and milk products are not the only sources of calcium. The chart on pages 21–22 lists non-dairy sources of calcium, such as almonds, sesame seeds, beans (especially soybeans, navy beans and chickpeas), "calcium greens" (greens containing calcium, such as broccoli, kale, napa cabbage, bok choy, collards) and tofu made with calcium sulfate or calcium chloride. These foods, together with canned salmon including the bones, canned sardines including the bones, lactose-free milk, yogurt, hard aged cheeses and fortified orange juice (with calcium) will be used in this cookbook to help you incorporate non-dairy sources of calcium into your diet.

The National Osteoporosis Foundation recommends 1,000 mg of calcium and 400 IU (International Units) of vitamin D per day for people aged 19 to 50, including pregnant and lactating women, and 1,500 mg of calcium and 800 IU of vitamin D per day for those over 50.

What Does Calcium Do for Us?

We need calcium to build strong bones and healthy teeth, for blood clotting and for the proper functioning of muscles, nerves and the heart. You will never outgrow the need for calcium, because bone matter is constantly being replaced by new bone.

We Cannot Produce Calcium Ourselves

We must eat foods that contain calcium; we then store calcium in our bodies for future use. If we do not eat enough foods containing calcium, our body automatically removes calcium stored in our bones and uses it to carry out the necessary bodily functions.

This constant "borrowing" from our calcium store can lead to a calcium deficiency that is further aggravated by the natural aging process. From about 35 onward, bone loss is likely to be a part of that process. This plus a calcium-deficient diet can result in fragile bones — a condition known as osteoporosis. This is a painful, disabling condition often affecting women after menopause (due to lack of estrogen), and men after the age of 60. It is essential that we have enough calcium in our stores prior to young adulthood to combat this process.

To reduce the risk of osteoporosis, we must:

- Get adequate vitamin D from the sun, food or a supplement (be sure to check with your doctor).
- Eat calcium-rich foods.
- Eat a varied diet, making sure to include choices from as many food groups as possible.
- Perform daily weight-bearing exercise, such as walking.
- Drink caffeine and alcohol in moderation.

Once you have been diagnosed by a doctor as lactose intolerant, it will be necessary to find your tolerance level to milk products in order to keep as many as possible in your daily diet. You can make up the difference with non-dairy sources of calcium (see chart on pages 21–22.)

You will notice that nutrition recommendations vary depending on your stage of life. For instance, rapidly growing children, pregnant women and nursing mothers all have high calcium needs. They must take in enough calcium for this additional growth so that their individual stores are not robbed of the mineral.

Protein and Calcium Absorption

In many countries where small amounts of protein are eaten and milk is not part of the diet, calcium is better utilized. The more protein ingested, the more calcium excreted by the body.

Bioavailability and Sources of Calcium

Bioavailability is the amount of a nutrient that can be absorbed and utilized by the body. For instance, the calcium from milk and milk products has excellent bioavailability — that is, most of the calcium consumed is used by the body. In contrast, there are a number of vegetables, such as spinach, beet greens and rhubarb, that are high in calcium but contain oxalic acid, which makes absorption of calcium in the small intestine difficult. Vegetables from the brassica family are oxalate-free and are a good source of calcium. These include kale, broccoli and bok choy.

Phytates are found in grains and legumes. They too make complete absorption of calcium difficult. Dietary fiber is also associated with reduced calcium absorption.

Surprising Soybeans

There are a number of nutritious foods made from soybeans. They are low in fat, cholesterol-free, easily digested, rich in protein and, in the case of tofu made with calcium sulfate or calcium chloride, a source of calcium. This is not news to people in Asian countries, but these foods are relatively new to us in North America (within the last hundred years).

Tofu

Tofu, also called soybean curd, is the vegetarian equivalent of cottage cheese in the dairy world. It is made by combining fresh hot soy milk with a coagulant to cause curdling. It is important to note for our purposes that if the coagulant used is calcium sulfate or calcium chloride, tofu becomes a source of calcium. It is also a cholesterol-free source of protein with unsaturated fat. To ensure that you are buying a tofu containing calcium, read the ingredient list on the label for the coagulant. Remember, it must read calcium chloride or calcium sulfate to be a calcium source.

Tofu can be high in fat; check the particular type you are using for fat content and use appropriately sized servings. Nevertheless, even though tofu contains fat, it is a lower-fat alternative to either sour cream or cream cheese, as the nutrient analysis comparison opposite shows. As you can see, tofu also contributes to protein. When coagulated with calcium chloride or calcium sulfate, it becomes a source of calcium too!

Compare: One Serving of	Old-Fashioned Chocolate Cheesecake made with cream cheese	Chocolate Cheesecake made with tofu
Calories	146.8	106.6
Protein	2.5 g	2.3 g
Carbohydrate	16.3 g	16.4 g
Fat	8.4 g	3.4 g
Calcium	20.7 mg	14.2 mg
Dietary Fiber	0.0 g	0.0 g
Percent of calories from:		
Carbohydrate	43%	59%
Protein	7%	8%
Fat	50%	32%

There are two types of tofu commonly available: cotton and silken

To make **cotton tofu**, soybean milk and the coagulant are combined in a cotton-lined container with holes. Weights are applied to the mixture to firm it up and press out the liquid. Cotton tofu is commonly found at the vegetable counters of supermarkets in soft, firm and extra-firm consistencies. Soft tofu is ideal for dressings, sauces and dips; firm tofu is good for cheesecake, puddings and spreads; and extra-firm is good for marinating, slicing, grilling and stir-frying.

Cotton tofu should be sold from a refrigerated counter like any fragile food. If it isn't, you will not be buying a product at its peak quality. When you get the tofu home, drain the liquid from it and cover it with fresh water. Re-cover and refrigerate. Packages are stamped with an expiry date and must be kept refrigerated; use the tofu by the expiry date listed on the package, changing the water daily.

Silken tofu is made from extra-thick soy milk. It is strained through silk (this process gives it the name "silken"), but the liquid is not drained off. The result is a creamy custard-like product. As with cotton tofu, soft silken tofu is ideal for dressings, sauces and dips; firm is good for cheesecake, puddings and spreads; and extra-firm is good for marinating, slicing, grilling and stir-frying.

Silken tofu is vacuum-packed and sometimes comes in convenient tetra packs or vacuum packed containers available at health food stores and some grocery stores. It has an expiry date stamped on the package but is shelf stable (if in the tetra pack) for several months; otherwise, refrigerate and use before the expiry date.

Soy Milk

Soy milk is the liquid squeezed from soaked soybeans. It has a beige color and a neutral flavor.

Soy milk can be purchased in supermarkets and health food stores, usually aseptically packed with an expiry date on the box. It is also known as soy beverage, and is sometimes labeled as such. It comes in a variety of flavors — plain, vanilla and chocolate are the most common.

Some stores may have fresh soy milk in a refrigerated section in bottles or cartons. Soy milk also comes powdered in boxes. Once rehydrated, it keeps for 5 days in the refrigerator.

As for its nutritional value, soy milk

- is now available fortified with calcium and vitamin D, essential for the absorption of calcium — be sure to check the label and purchase the fortified variety
- has about the same amount of fat as cow's milk, and is also available in 1%
- is rich in protein
- is rich in iron
- is cholesterol-free
- is low in saturated fat
- is lactose-free

Soy milk should not be used for infants. They require a specially prepared commercial soy-based infant formula to fill their nutritional needs.

Tips on Using Tofu and Soy Milk in Recipes

1. Tofu needs to be drained in a sieve before it is added to a recipe.

2. Tofu and soy milk both have a bland, flat flavor. When I worked with them in the recipes, I found it necessary to add more spices or herbs than I would have if I had been using a milk product. If you try to adapt some of your own recipes, remember that you cannot substitute soy milk or tofu directly for milk or milk products and expect exactly the same taste results. The soy foods seem to absorb flavorings. However, once additional flavoring is added, the recipe should be tasty.

3. In the case of soy milk, it may be necessary to add ingredients with more color or to add a garnish to compensate for the beige color of the dishes.

4. Because it is a convenient, shelf-stable product and has a delicate texture and flavor, silken tofu is an excellent substitute for sour cream and cream cheese in cheesecake, dips and spreads. Again, added seasoning is required to compensate for the bland taste. Experiment with the different kinds of tofu yourself to see what works best for you.

5. Use extra-firm tofu to replace meat: it keeps its shape while cooking and has a texture more similar to meat than does softer tofu. Because tofu is bland in flavor, it is often marinated before cooking. Like meat, tofu can be browned in hot oil first, then cooked on medium or low heat to simmer and absorb the flavors of the dish.

6. For a smooth texture, use a food processor or blender to purée soft tofu. This is particularly important in dressings or sauces where a silky consistency is required.

7. Leftover tofu can be wrapped carefully and frozen for up to 6 months. The texture will change, but it will make a chewy meat-like substitute for ground meat or crumbled cheese. Defrost the tofu in the refrigerator for 24 hours. Squeeze out moisture before using.

Getting Enough Calcium

Dairy products are an excellent source of calcium. North American food guides recommend that we consume milk and milk products on a daily basis for both calcium and vitamin D (remember that vitamin D is essential for the absorption of calcium). But that doesn't mean the lactose-intolerant person must rely on calcium supplements. The food we eat can be a much better source of calcium than supplements. By carefully choosing dairy foods that are easier for those with lactose intolerance to digest and by including non-dairy foods that are rich in calcium and vitamin D, it is possible to consume the recommended amount of calcium without supplements.

The current recommended dietary intake (RDI) of calcium is as follows: children age 4 to 8, 800 mg/day; adolescents age 9 to 18, 1,300 mg/day; adults age 19 to 50 (including pregnant and lactating women), 1,000 mg/day; adults over 50, 1,200 to 1,500 mg/day.

Here are some ideas to help you increase the calcium in your diet:

- Buy lactose-free milk.

- Try drinking or cooking with milk in small quantities, $\frac{1}{4}$ cup (50 mL) at a time.

- Eat small quantities of hard aged cheese, such as Parmesan or aged Cheddar. Start small and build up to the quantity you can tolerate.

- Try eating and cooking with yogurt: the bacteria in yogurt helps break down lactose; thus, it is more easily digested than many dairy products.

- Buy lactase tablets, available over the counter at pharmacies (you will usually have to ask the pharmacist for a bottle). Taken before you eat lactose-containing foods, they help you digest the lactose in your system.

- Include fortified soy milk and calcium-fortified fruit juices in your daily diet.

- Include a variety of calcium-containing non-dairy foods in your daily diet (see the chart on pages 21–22 to learn how much calcium these foods contain).

For all age groups, the RDI of vitamin D is 400 to 800 IU a day, with adults over 50 needing the most. In addition to fattier fish sources such as salmon, vitamin D is added to margarine and milk. Check with your physician or dietitian to see if your intake of vitamin D is adequate.

Dietary choices should go hand in hand with the other necessary component for healthy bones: exercise. Weight-bearing exercise of 30 minutes or more at least 3 times a week is considered necessary for maintaining good bone health.

Approximate Calcium Content of Some Common Foods

Item	Portion	Calcium (mg)
MILK, MILK PRODUCTS, MILK SUBSTITUTE		
Milk (skim, 1%, 2%, homogenized)	1 cup (250 mL)	300
Buttermilk and chocolate milk	1 cup (250 mL)	285
Fortified soy milk	1 cup (250 mL)	300
Evaporated milk, undiluted	$\frac{1}{2}$ cup (125 mL)	350
Instant skim milk powder	3 tbsp (45 mL)	155
Ice cream	$\frac{1}{2}$ cup (125 mL)	80
Light sour cream	1 tbsp (15 mL)	30
Sour cream	1 tbsp (15 mL)	15
Plain yogurt	$\frac{3}{4}$ cup (175 g)	300
Fruit yogurt	$\frac{3}{4}$ cup (175 g)	250
Swiss cheese	$1\frac{3}{4}$ oz (50 g)	480
Light Cheddar cheese	$1\frac{3}{4}$ oz (50 g)	385
Cheddar cheese	$1\frac{3}{4}$ oz (50 g)	360
Grated Parmesan cheese	1 tbsp (15 mL)	85
Cream cheese	1 tbsp (15 mL)	12
Ricotta cheese	$\frac{1}{2}$ cup (125 mL)	255
Light ricotta cheese	$\frac{1}{2}$ cup (125 mL)	335
Cottage cheese	$\frac{1}{2}$ cup (125 mL)	75
MEAT, FISH, POULTRY, ALTERNATIVES		
Salmon including bones, canned, drained	Half $7\frac{1}{2}$ oz (213 g) can	225
Sardines including bones, 8 small, drained	$\frac{1}{2}$ oz (15 g)	165
Tuna, canned, drained	Half $7\frac{1}{2}$ oz (213 g) can	23
Turkey, dark meat, roasted, no skin	3 oz (90 g)	27
Turkey, light meat, roasted, no skin	3 oz (90 g)	16
Chicken, light or dark meat, roasted, no skin	3 oz (90 g)	13
Egg	1 large	24
Pork, roasted, lean only	3 oz (90 g)	24
Lamb, roasted, lean only	3 oz (90 g)	12
Beef, roasted, lean only	3 oz (90 g)	8
SHELLFISH		
Clams, canned, drained	$\frac{1}{2}$ cup (125 mL)	75
Shrimp, canned, drained	$\frac{1}{2}$ cup (125 mL)	40
Crab, canned, drained	$\frac{1}{2}$ cup (125 mL)	28
Mussels, cooked	2 medium	25
Oysters, raw	2 medium	10
LEGUMES AND TOFU		
Soybeans, canned or boiled	1 cup (250 mL)	175
Baked beans, canned or boiled	1 cup (250 mL)	150
Navy beans, canned or boiled	1 cup (250 mL)	125
Pinto beans, canned or boiled	1 cup (250 mL)	85
Chickpeas, canned or boiled	1 cup (250 mL)	75

Item	Portion	Calcium (mg)
Kidney beans, canned or boiled	1 cup (250 mL)	55
Tofu, containing 10% of Recommended Daily Intake of calcium per 90 g*	½ cup (125 mL) cubed (3 oz/90 g)	110

NUTS AND SEEDS

Item	Portion	Calcium (mg)
Almonds	½ cup (125 mL)	190
Hazelnuts	½ cup (125 mL)	130
Sesame seeds	½ cup (125 mL)	100
Walnuts	½ cup (125 mL)	45
Pecans	½ cup (125 mL)	20

BAKING INGREDIENTS

Item	Portion	Calcium (mg)
Soy flour	1 cup (250 mL)	240
All-purpose flour	1 cup (250 mL)	20
Blackstrap molasses	2 tbsp (25 mL)	280
Fancy molasses	2 tbsp (25 mL)	70

PASTA (weight and measure before cooking)

Item	Portion	Calcium (mg)
Soy pasta (e.g., ¾ cup/175 mL macaroni)	3 oz (90 g)	24
Regular pasta (e.g., ¾ cup/175 mL macaroni)	3 oz (90 g)	16

BAKING INGREDIENTS

Item	Portion	Calcium (mg)
White bread	1 slice	20
Whole wheat bread	1 slice	24

FRUIT

Item	Portion	Calcium (mg)
Figs, dried, chopped	½ cup (125 mL)	120
Currants, dried, chopped	½ cup (125 mL)	60
Raisins	½ cup (125 mL)	40
Apricots, dried, chopped	½ cup (125 mL)	30
Dates, dried, chopped	½ cup (125 mL)	30
Oranges, whole, fresh	1 medium	50

VEGETABLES**

Item	Portion	Calcium (mg)
Bok choy, shredded, raw	½ cup (125 mL)	35
Bok choy, shredded, cooked	½ cup (125 mL)	80
Broccoli, chopped, raw	½ cup (125 mL)	20
Broccoli, chopped, cooked	½ cup (125 mL)	35
Cabbage, shredded, raw	½ cup (125 mL)	15
Cabbage, shredded, cooked	½ cup (125 mL)	25
Collards, chopped, cooked	½ cup (125 mL)	15
Kale, chopped, raw	½ cup (125 mL)	45
Mustard greens, chopped, cooked	½ cup (125 mL)	52
Napa cabbage, shredded, raw	½ cup (125 mL)	30
Turnip greens, chopped, raw	½ cup (125 mL)	105

*On labels, calcium content is expressed as a percentage of Recommended Daily Intake (%RDI). To determine calcium content in mg, multiply %RDI by 1,100.

**A volume of cooked vegetables (e.g., ½ cup/125 mL) will have a higher calcium content than the same quantity of raw; the change in texture resulting from cooking means more vegetables can be packed in.

Dips, Spreads and Other Nibbles

Your dipping days are not over if you are lactose intolerant. Typically, appetizers use cream cheese and sour cream as a base. Silken soft and firm tofu can play a major role in replacing these lactose products, with excellent results. No one will know the difference!

Tofu tastes bland and absorbs flavors. By adding more herbs and spices than you would when using cream cheese or sour cream, you can compensate for this. Make sure you taste as you are working with the tofu in a recipe, and note your preferences of seasonings as you go along.

A food processor is a real asset because it can turn tofu into a smooth, creamy dip that would otherwise be lumpy. If a food processor is not available, use an electric mixer or blender. These appetizers are easy to digest and are lighter than the original versions because tofu has a lower fat content than cream cheese or sour cream.

Shelf-stable silken tofu, available from the health food store, has definitely become a staple in my pantry!

Creamy Veggie Dip 24

Tex-Mex Bean and Salsa
    Pyramid Dip. 25

Sun Dried Tomato and
    Parsley Pesto Dip 26

Soybean Hummus 28

Guacamole Spread. 29

Double Salmon Spread. 30

Smoked Salmon Pâté. 31

Seafood Pâté 32

Herbed Pâté 33

Salsa. 34

Tortilla Chips 35

Nachos with Beans 36

Mexican Tortilla Rolls 37

Antojitos. 38

Pitas Stuffed with Hummus
    and Sprouts. 39

Mediterranean Crostini 40

Spanakopita 42

Kale Tart with Sun-Dried Tomatoes
    and Pine Nuts 44

Mushroom Strudel. 46

Cocktail Crunch 48

Salted Almonds. 49

Dried Fruit with Goat Cheese. 50

Creamy Veggie Dip

Many sour cream– and cream cheese–based dips served with crudités are taboo for the lactose intolerant. But you won't miss those ingredients with this yummy dip.

TIPS

To reduce fat, use light mayonnaise.

If fresh tarragon is not available, use 1 tbsp (15 mL) dried.

MAKE AHEAD

Spoon into an airtight container and store in the refrigerator for up to 2 days.

2	green onions, chopped	2
1	clove garlic, minced	1
2 cups	light mayonnaise	500 mL
1/4 cup	chopped fresh parsley	50 mL
2 tbsp	minced fresh tarragon	25 mL
2 tbsp	freshly squeezed lemon juice	25 mL
1/2 tsp	salt	2 mL
1/4 tsp	freshly ground black pepper	1 mL

1. In a food processor, using pulsing action, purée green onions, garlic, mayonnaise, parsley, tarragon, lemon juice, salt and pepper.

Variation

Experiment with a variety of herbs, such as basil and thyme.

Nutritional value
Per serving (2 tbsp/25 mL)

Calories	76
Protein	0 g
Fat	6 g
Carbohydrate	5 g
Dietary Fiber	0 g
Calcium	6 mg

Percent of calories from

Protein	2%
Fat	71%
Carbohydrate	27%

Tex-Mex Bean and Salsa Pyramid Dip

This versatile recipe can be used as an appetizer for a casual party, or as a main course salad or accompaniment to a barbecue. Use the tortilla chips to scoop up all the delectable mixture. Guacamole Spread (see recipe, page 29) can replace the tofu mixture for a different taste.

MAKES ABOUT 10 SERVINGS

TIP

Check ingredient list on tortilla chips for milk solids before buying.

MAKE AHEAD

Cover and store in the refrigerator for up to 4 hours.

1	package (10.25 oz/290 g) silken soft tofu	1
5 cups	shredded lettuce	1.25 L
1 cup	sunflower or alfalfa sprouts	250 mL
2 tbsp	light mayonnaise	25 mL
2 tbsp	freshly squeezed lemon juice	25 mL
1 cup	salsa	250 mL
1	can (19 oz/540 mL) kidney beans, drained	1
¾ cup	sliced black olives	175 mL
½ cup	chopped red bell pepper	125 mL
2	green onions, chopped	2
	Tortilla chips	

1. Using a sieve, drain tofu.
2. Arrange lettuce and sprouts in single layer on a 12-inch (30 cm) round platter.
3. In a food processor, beat together drained tofu, mayonnaise and lemon juice until smooth. Spread on top of lettuce, leaving a 1-inch (2.5 cm) border.
4. Spread salsa on top, leaving a 1-inch (2.5 cm) border. Sprinkle kidney beans on top of salsa. Pile olives in center. Surround olives with a ring of red pepper. Surround red pepper with ring of onions. Serve with tortilla chips.

Nutritional value
Per serving

Calories	145
Protein	6 g
Fat	7 g
Carbohydrate	16 g
Dietary Fiber (a high source)	4 g
Calcium (a source)	79 mg

Percent of calories from

Protein	16%
Fat	42%
Carbohydrate	42%

Sun-Dried Tomato and Parsley Pesto Dip

Serve with sliced baguette and assorted vegetables. Remember to include calcium carriers such as broccoli and kale! You can substitute ½ cup (125 mL) prepared pesto for the homemade.

MAKES ABOUT 2 CUPS (500 ML)

MAKE AHEAD

Spoon into an airtight container and store in the refrigerator for up to 2 days.

8 oz	soft tofu, drained	250 g
6	drained whole sun-dried tomatoes, packed in oil	6
1	clove garlic, minced	1
½ cup	Parsley Pesto (see recipe, opposite)	125 mL

1. Using a sieve, drain tofu.
2. In a food processor, using pulsing action, combine tofu, sun-dried tomatoes, garlic and pesto; purée until almost smooth.

Dry-packed sun-dried tomatoes are cheaper than those packed in oil. To rehydrate, cover with boiling water and simmer for about 5 minutes. Drain and cover with extra-virgin olive oil and minced garlic clove. Transfer to a jar and refrigerate for up to 1 week.

Tofu can successfully replace cream cheese in many recipes. To compensate for tofu's bland taste, you may need to use a little more salt, lemon juice and herbs to give the mixture more zip. Tofu, a protein and iron source, is lactose-free, and if it is coagulated with calcium sulfate or calcium chloride, it is a calcium source lower in fat than cream cheese.

Nutritional value
Per serving (2 tbsp/25 mL)

Calories	41
Protein	2 g
Fat	3 g
Carbohydrate	1 g
Dietary Fiber	0 g
Calcium	35 mg

Percent of calories from

Protein	18%
Fat	64%
Carbohydrate	18%

Parsley Pesto

MAKES ½ CUP (125 ML)

1 cup	fresh parsley leaves, washed and dried	250 mL
2 tbsp	grated Parmesan cheese (optional, if tolerated)	25 mL
1 tbsp	toasted pine nuts	15 mL
1 tbsp	dried basil	15 mL
1	large clove garlic	1
½ tsp	salt	2 mL
¼ tsp	freshly ground black pepper	1 mL
¼ cup	extra-virgin olive oil	50 mL

MAKE AHEAD

Spoon into an airtight container and store in the refrigerator for up to 2 weeks or in the freezer for up to 4 months. Be sure to freeze in a convenient size, such as ¼-cup (50 mL) portions.

1. In a food processor, combine parsley, cheese (if using), pine nuts, basil, garlic, salt and pepper until finely chopped. With motor running, pour in oil through feed tube and beat until well combined.

Soybean Hummus

Hummus is a Middle Eastern spread traditionally made with chickpeas. Although chickpeas contain some calcium, soybeans and navy beans contain more. For convenience, use canned soybeans, navy beans or chickpeas, available in some supermarkets and health food stores.

MAKES ABOUT 2 CUPS (500 ML)

TIPS

For added calcium, serve with sesame crackers or Tortilla Chips (see recipe, page 35).

One lemon yields about ¼ cup (50 mL) juice.

MAKE AHEAD

Spoon into an airtight container and store in the refrigerator for up to 3 days.

2	green onions, chopped	2
1	clove garlic, crushed	1
1	can (19 oz/540 mL) soybeans, navy beans or chickpeas, drained and rinsed	1
¼ cup	chopped fresh parsley	50 mL
¼ cup	freshly squeezed lemon juice	50 mL
¼ cup	olive oil	50 mL
¼ tsp	salt	1 mL
¼ tsp	freshly ground black pepper	1 mL

1. In a food processor, using pulsing action, purée green onions, garlic, soybeans, parsley, lemon juice, olive oil, salt and pepper.

Nutritional value
Per serving (2 tbsp/25 mL)

Calories	71
Protein	4 g
Fat	5 g
Carbohydrate	3 g
Dietary Fiber	1 g
Calcium	29 mg

Percent of calories from

Protein	19%
Fat	63%
Carbohydrate	19%

Guacamole Spread

Dip tortilla or corn chips into this zesty spread or serve a dollop over sliced tomatoes. It is the perfect companion to chicken salad, whether in a sandwich or in a pita with sprouts. You can keep the spread covered and refrigerated for up to two days.

MAKES ABOUT 1½ CUPS (375 ML)

TIP

If an avocado is ripe, it will give slightly to pressure without feeling mushy. The skin will be brownish green rather than bright green. If only hard, under-ripe avocados are available, buy in advance and store in a paper bag or with a bunch of bananas to hasten ripening.

MAKE AHEAD

Spoon into an airtight container and store in the refrigerator for up to 2 days.

1	package (10.25 oz/290 g) silken soft tofu	1
1	ripe avocado, peeled and pitted	1
2 tbsp	freshly squeezed lemon juice	25 mL
1 tbsp	vegetable oil	15 mL
2 tsp	Dijon mustard	10 mL
1 tsp	salt	5 mL
1 tsp	granulated sugar	5 mL
¼ tsp	freshly ground black pepper	1 mL
Pinch	cayenne pepper	Pinch

1. Using a sieve, drain tofu.
2. In a food processor, purée drained tofu, avocado, lemon juice, oil, mustard, salt, sugar, black pepper and cayenne pepper until smooth.

Nutritional value
Per serving (1 tbsp/15 mL)

Calories	24
Protein	1 g
Fat	2 g
Carbohydrate	1 g
Dietary Fiber	0 g
Calcium	5 mg

Percent of calories from

Protein	11%
Fat	71%
Carbohydrate	18%

Double Salmon Spread

Don't forget to include the salmon bones for a calcium boost in this spread. Serve on melba toast, garnished with a sprig of dill.

MAKES ABOUT 1 CUP (250 ML)

MAKE AHEAD

Spoon into an airtight container and store in the refrigerator for up to 2 days.

1	package (10.25 oz/290 g) silken soft tofu	1
1	can (7.5 oz/213 g) sockeye salmon	1
4 oz	smoked salmon	125 g
1/4 cup	fresh dill sprigs	50 mL
1/4 cup	freshly squeezed lemon juice	50 mL
2 tbsp	light mayonnaise	25 mL
2 tbsp	chopped green onion	25 mL
1 tsp	horseradish	5 mL
1/4 tsp	freshly ground black pepper	1 mL

1. Using a sieve, drain tofu. Drain sockeye salmon; discard skin and dark pieces, reserving bones.

2. In a food processor, using pulsing action, combine drained tofu, salmon with bones, smoked salmon, dill, lemon juice, mayonnaise, onion, horseradish and pepper until smooth.

Nutritional value
Per serving (1 tbsp/15 mL)

Calories	45
Protein	4 g
Fat	3 g
Carbohydrate	1 g
Dietary Fiber	0 g
Calcium	46 mg

Percent of calories from

Protein	39%
Fat	50%
Carbohydrate	11%

Smoked Salmon Pâté

This elegant pâté, based on the original recipe with oodles of cream, has no cream!
It makes a great party appetizer: Garnish with lemon slices and serve with crackers.

MAKES ABOUT 4 CUPS (1 L)

TIP

This is your chance to use that fancy mold you've been storing. If you don't have one, use a loaf pan lined with plastic wrap instead.

MAKE AHEAD

Store in the refrigerator for up to 1 day.

Nutritional value
Per serving (1 tbsp/15 mL)

Calories	12
Protein	2 g
Fat	1 g
Carbohydrate	0 g
Dietary Fiber	0 g
Calcium	2 mg

Percent of calories from

Protein	49%
Fat	42%
Carbohydrate	9%

● *4-cup (1 L) mold, lined with plastic wrap*

1	package (10.25 oz/290 g) silken soft tofu	1
1	envelope (1/4 oz/7 g) unflavored gelatin	1
1/4 cup	water, at room temperature	50 mL
12 oz	smoked salmon	375 g
1/4 cup	light mayonnaise	50 mL
2 tbsp	freshly squeezed lemon juice	25 mL
1/4 tsp	freshly ground black pepper	1 mL
3	egg whites	3

1. Using a sieve, drain tofu.

2. In a small saucepan, sprinkle gelatin over water. Set aside.

3. In a food processor, using pulsing action, combine drained tofu, salmon, mayonnaise, lemon juice and pepper until smooth.

4. Dissolve gelatin over medium heat for about 3 minutes, or until clear. With motor of food processor running, pour gelatin through feed tube and beat until well combined.

5. In a large bowl, using an electric mixer, beat egg whites on high speed until stiff peaks form. Spoon into salmon mixture. Using pulsing action, combine just until no white shows.

6. Spoon salmon mixture into prepared mold. Cover and refrigerate for at least 2 hours, until set.

7. Place a serving plate over mold. Invert mold and, using plastic wrap as a lever, unmold onto plate. Discard plastic wrap. Smooth pâté surface with knife.

> This recipe contains raw egg whites. If the food safety of raw eggs is a concern for you, use pasteurized eggs in their shells.

Seafood Pâté

This makes a flavorful sandwich filling or party spread for tortillas. For tortilla spirals, simply spread seafood pâté on tortillas, roll up tightly jelly-roll fashion in plastic wrap, twisting ends and tucking under. Refrigerate until an hour or two before serving, then slice in 2-inch (5 cm) pieces. For best flavor, buy fresh shrimp and cook them for this recipe.

MAKES ABOUT 4 CUPS (1 L)

TIP

Lemon juice from freshly squeezed lemons gives a flavor superior to bottled concentrate. To get the most juice out of your lemons, let them stand at room temperature to warm up or immerse in hot water for a minute.

MAKE AHEAD

Spoon into an airtight container and store in the refrigerator for up to 2 days.

1	package (10.25 oz/290 g) silken soft tofu	1
2	cans (each 7.5 oz/213 g) sockeye salmon	2
4 oz	cooked fresh shrimp	125 g
1/4 cup	light mayonnaise	50 mL
2 tbsp	freshly squeezed lemon juice	25 mL
1 tbsp	ketchup	15 mL
1 tbsp	grated onion	15 mL
1 tsp	Worcestershire sauce	5 mL
Dash	hot pepper sauce	Dash

1. Using a sieve, drain tofu. Drain salmon; discard skin and dark pieces, reserving bones.

2. In a food processor, using pulsing action, combine drained tofu, salmon with bones, shrimp, mayonnaise, lemon juice, ketchup, onion, Worcestershire sauce and hot pepper sauce until smooth.

Nutritional value
Per serving (1 tbsp/15 mL)

Calories	17
Protein	2 g
Fat	1 g
Carbohydrate	0 g
Dietary Fiber	0 g
Calcium	17 mg

Percent of calories from

Protein	40%
Fat	52%
Carbohydrate	8%

Herbed Pâté

Silken soft tofu replaces the original recipe's sour cream and cream cheese with less fat, and it provides calcium if made with calcium chloride. Be sure to check the ingredient list on the label for calcium chloride or calcium sulfate. This creamy, garlicky concoction takes minutes to make in a food processor. Serve with a medley of crudités. Be sure to include broccoli and strips of bok choy as a calcium source.

MAKES ABOUT 1⅓ CUPS (325 ML)

MAKE AHEAD

Store in the refrigerator for up to 2 days.

1	package (10.25 oz/290 g) silken soft tofu	1
2	green onions, chopped	2
1	clove garlic, minced	1
½ cup	chopped fresh parsley	125 mL
2 tbsp	light mayonnaise	25 mL
2 tbsp	freshly squeezed lemon juice	25 mL
2 tbsp	chopped green olives	25 mL
1 tsp	Worcestershire sauce	5 mL
½ tsp	salt	2 ml
¼ tsp	dried thyme	1 mL
¼ tsp	freshly ground black pepper	1 mL
Dash	hot pepper sauce	Dash

1. Using a sieve, drain tofu.
2. In a food processor, using pulsing action, combine drained tofu, onions, garlic, parsley, mayonnaise, lemon juice, olives, Worcestershire sauce, salt, thyme, pepper and hot pepper sauce until well blended.
3. Spoon into a serving bowl. For best flavor, cover and refrigerate for 1 day.

Nutritional value
Per serving (1 tbsp/15 mL)

Calories	13
Protein	1 g
Fat	1 g
Carbohydrate	1 g
Dietary Fiber	0 g
Calcium	8 mg

Percent of calories from

Protein	22%
Fat	52%
Carbohydrate	26%

Salsa

This quickly concocted, spicy, fresh relish is ideal to make when tomatoes are at their juicy best.

MAKE AHEAD

Cover and let stand at room temperature for up to 2 hours.

2	tomatoes, chopped	2
2	cloves garlic, minced	2
½	green bell pepper, chopped	½
¼ cup	chopped green onion	50 mL
2 tbsp	chopped fresh cilantro	25 mL
1 tbsp	chopped jalapeño pepper	15 mL
1 tbsp	freshly squeezed lime juice	15 mL
1 tbsp	olive oil	15 mL
1 tsp	red wine vinegar	5 mL
½ tsp	salt	2 mL
Pinch	freshly ground black pepper	Pinch

1. In a medium bowl, stir together tomatoes, garlic, green pepper, green onion, cilantro, jalapeño pepper, lime juice, oil, vinegar, salt and pepper.

Nutritional value
Per serving (1 tbsp/15 mL)

Calories	6
Protein	0 g
Fat	0 g
Carbohydrate	0 g
Dietary Fiber	0 g
Calcium	2 mg

Percent of calories from

Protein	6%
Fat	64%
Carbohydrate	30%

Tortilla Chips

A few packaged tortilla wraps can be transformed into these delectable crunchy flat breads, ideal for serving with a dip or spread. Be generous with the sesame seeds, as they are a source of calcium.

TIPS

This is a great way to recycle stale wraps.

Egg white acts as an edible glue in baking.

MAKE AHEAD

Place in a cookie tin and store at room temperature for up to 1 day. (However, they are best the day they are made.)

Nutritional value
Per serving (1 dozen)

Calories	156
Protein	5 g
Fat	7 g
Carbohydrate	19 g
Dietary Fiber (a source)	2 g
Calcium (a source)	128 mg

Percent of calories from

Protein	12%
Fat	41%
Carbohydrate	47%

● *Preheat oven to 350°F (180°C)*
● *Baking sheet, lined with parchment paper*

4	10-inch (25 cm) flour tortillas	4
1	egg white, beaten	1
¼ cup	sesame seeds	50 mL

1. Using a pastry brush, lightly brush each tortilla with egg white and sprinkle with sesame seeds. Stack tortillas and, using a sharp chef's knife, cut tortillas into 12 equal wedges.

2. Arrange wedges in a single layer on prepared baking sheet. Bake in preheated oven for 10 to 13 minutes, or until a deep golden brown.

Variation

For variety, use flavored wraps or pitas with a combination of sesame seeds and poppy seeds.

Nachos with Beans

A kid-friendly recipe, this quick adaptation is ideal for the lactose intolerant.

TIP

This is great, simple entertaining fare. Make sure to provide abundant napkins!

1	recipe Tortilla Chips (page 35)	1
1	recipe New-Fashioned Bean Pot (page 174)	1
1 cup	salsa	250 mL
2 cups	shredded old Cheddar cheese (optional, if tolerated)	500 mL
½	head shredded lettuce	125 mL

1. Prepare Tortilla Chips and New-Fashioned Bean Pot as indicated in the recipes.

2. On a large tray, arrange ingredients in concentric circles, starting in the center with the bean pot and going outward: bean pot, salsa, cheese (if using) and lettuce and tortilla chips.

Variation

If you prefer, use nacho chips instead of homemade tortilla chips.

Nutritional value
Per serving

Calories	436
Protein	18 g
Fat	20 g
Carbohydrate	46 g
Dietary Fiber (a very high source)	10 g
Calcium (a very high source)	406 mg

Percent of calories from

Protein	17%
Fat	41%
Carbohydrate	42%

Mexican Tortilla Rolls

These colorful sandwiches are popular with all ages. Serve with bowls of Salsa (see recipe, page 34) and Tofu Cream (see recipe, page 247) for dipping.

(see recipe, page 34) and Tofu Cream (see recipe, page 247)

MAKES ABOUT 20 PIECES

TIPS

Leftover tofu can be wrapped and frozen. Although crumbly in texture when defrosted, the tofu can be used in dishes such as chili to replace or supplement meat.

The firmer the tofu, the higher the fat, protein and calcium content.

MAKE AHEAD

Store in the refrigerator for up to 1 day.

Nutritional value
Per serving (1 piece)

Calories	42
Protein	1 g
Fat	2 g
Carbohydrate	5 g
Dietary Fiber	1 g
Calcium	28 mg

Percent of calories from

Protein	12%
Fat	40%
Carbohydrate	48%

Filling

2	green onions, chopped	2
6 oz	extra-firm tofu, crumbled	175 g
3/4 cup	salsa	175 mL
1/2 cup	sliced black olives	125 mL
1/2 cup	chopped red bell pepper	125 mL
1/3 cup	chopped fresh coriander	75 mL
1 tsp	grated lime zest	5 mL
2 tbsp	freshly squeezed lime juice	25 mL
1/2 tsp	salt	2 mL
4	10-inch (25 cm) flour tortillas	4

1. *Prepare the filling:* In food processor, using pulsing motion, combine onions, tofu, salsa, olives, red pepper, coriander, lime zest, lime juice and salt.

2. Spread about 1/2 cup (125 mL) filling on each tortilla, leaving a 1/2-inch (1 cm) border.

3. Roll up tightly and wrap in plastic wrap. Refrigerate for at least 1 hour to allow flavors to mellow and to firm up for easy slicing.

4. To serve, unwrap and slice 5 diagonal pieces about 2 inches (10 cm) long. Discard trimmings.

Antojitos

A popular Mexican-style snack, these can be made as hot as you like, depending on the peppers used in the recipe.

MAKES ABOUT 24 PIECES

TIP

The general rule for peppers is, the smaller the pepper, the hotter the taste. Jalapeño peppers are small, green, cone-shaped peppers that are much hotter than the large red, green, yellow or orange bell peppers. They are usually carefully labeled in supermarkets, but if in doubt, ask!

Nutritional value
Per serving (1 piece)

Calories	33
Protein	1 g
Fat	2 g
Carbohydrate	4 g
Dietary Fiber	0 g
Calcium	16 mg

Percent of calories from

Protein	15%
Fat	41%
Carbohydrate	44%

● Baking sheet

Filling

1	package (10.5 oz/297 g) silken firm tofu	1
1 tbsp	vegetable oil	15 mL
½ tsp	salt	2 mL
½ tsp	granulated sugar	2 mL
¼ cup	chopped red bell pepper	50 mL
¼ cup	chopped jalapeño peppers	50 mL
2 tbsp	chopped black olives	25 mL
4	10-inch (25 cm) flour tortillas	4
	Salsa (store-bought or see recipe, page 34)	

1. *Prepare the filling:* Using a sieve, drain tofu.

2. In a food processor, purée drained tofu, oil, salt and sugar until smooth. Stir in red pepper, jalapeño peppers and olives just until combined.

3. Spread each tortilla with about ⅓ cup (75 mL) filling, leaving a 1-inch (2.5 cm) border. Roll up and wrap tightly in plastic wrap. Refrigerate for at least 1 hour or for up to 4 hours.

4. Preheat oven to 350°F (180°C). Cut antojitos into 1½-inch (4 cm) pieces and arrange on baking sheet.

5. Bake for about 10 minutes, or until heated through. Serve immediately with salsa for dipping.

Pitas Stuffed with Hummus and Sprouts

Making these bite-size pockets with sprouts, tahini and white kidney beans enhances the calcium content. Hummus can be made in minutes in the food processor. It's great in a pita pocket, but it's yummy with crudités too.

MAKES 20 PIECES

TIPS

White kidney beans and sesame seeds are alternative sources of calcium. See page 22.

Tahini is available in the specialty section of supermarkets and in Middle Eastern food stores.

MAKE AHEAD

Cover and store in the refrigerator for up to 8 hours.

Nutritional value
Per serving (1 piece)

Calories	55
Protein	3 g
Fat	1 g
Carbohydrate	10 g
Dietary Fiber (a source)	3 g
Calcium	17 mg

Percent of calories from

Protein	19%
Fat	14%
Carbohydrate	66%

4	green onions	4
1	clove garlic, minced	1
1	can (19 oz/540 mL) white kidney beans, drained	1
½ cup	loosely packed fresh parsley leaves	125 mL
¼ cup	freshly squeezed lemon juice	50 mL
2 tbsp	tahini	25 mL
¼ tsp	freshly ground black pepper	1 mL
20	whole wheat cocktail pitas (about 1 package)	20
1½ cups	sunflower or alfalfa sprouts	375 mL

1. In a food processor, using pulsing action, combine onions, garlic, beans, parsley, lemon juice, tahini and pepper.

2. Using a sharp knife, cut halfway around seams of pitas. Spoon a generous 1 tbsp (15 mL) hummus into each pita; top with about 1 tbsp (15 mL) sprouts.

Mediterranean Crostini

This speedy snack is ideal as a simple appetizer or as an accompaniment to soup or salad for a light meal. Sardines add extra zip and calcium to the topping. Although you can use a commercial tomato sauce for added speed, this flavorful homemade tomato sauce is quick and easy — and too good to miss.

MAKES ABOUT 35 PIECES

TIP

If cheese is not tolerated, crumble firm tofu or defrosted frozen tofu over crostini.

MAKE AHEAD

Prepare through Step 2, cover and refrigerate for up to 3 hours.

● *Baking sheet*

1	baguette (16 inches/40 cm long), cut into ½ inch (1 cm) thick slices	1
2 cups	Homemade Tomato Sauce (see recipe, opposite) or store-bought thick tomato pasta sauce	500 mL
1	can (3¾ oz/100 g) sardines, drained and patted dry	1
1 cup	freshly grated Parmesan cheese (optional, if tolerated)	250 mL

1. Spread each slice of baguette with about 1 tbsp (15 mL) Homemade Tomato Sauce.

2. Coarsely chop sardines; place 1 piece on center of each slice. Sprinkle with cheese (if using). Arrange on baking sheet.

3. Preheat oven to 375°F (190°C). Bake crostini for about 5 minutes or until heated through. Serve immediately.

Nutritional value
Per serving (1 piece)

Calories	61
Protein	3 g
Fat	3 g
Carbohydrate	8 g
Dietary Fiber	1 g
Calcium (a source)	71 mg

Percent of calories from

Protein	21%
Fat	30%
Carbohydrate	49%

Homemade Tomato Sauce

2 tbsp	extra-virgin olive oil	25 mL
2	cloves garlic, minced	2
1 cup	finely chopped onions	250 mL
1	can (28 oz/796 mL) tomatoes, drained and chopped	1
1	can (5 1/2 oz/156 mL) tomato paste	1
2 tbsp	freshly squeezed lemon juice	25 mL
1 tsp	dried basil	5 mL
1 tsp	dried oregano	5 mL
1/2 tsp	granulated sugar	2 mL
1/2 tsp	salt	2 mL
	Freshly ground black pepper	
1/4 cup	chopped fresh parsley	50 mL

MAKE AHEAD

Spoon into an airtight container and store in the refrigerator for up to 1 day or in the freezer for up to 6 months (be sure to label and date the container).

1. In a large saucepan, heat oil over medium-high heat. Add garlic and onions; cook, covered, until onions are softened, about 5 minutes.

2. Stir in tomatoes, tomato paste, lemon juice, basil, oregano, sugar and salt; cook until sauce is heated through and thickened, about 5 minutes. Season with pepper to taste. Stir in parsley.

Spanakopita

These crispy Greek-style triangles are traditionally made with a spinach and cheese mixture, but tofu replaces cheese in this lactose-free version. Kale, similar in taste to spinach but a better calcium source, can be substituted for spinach. (See Braised Kale on page 162 for preparation instructions.)

MAKES ABOUT 24 PIECES

TIPS

If a full bunch of dill, parsley or any other fresh herb is more than you need for a recipe, wash, dry and chop whatever is left over, wrap it in plastic wrap, label it and freeze it for up to 1 year. It's the ultimate convenience for future recipes.

One half lemon will yield about 2 tbsp (25 mL) of juice, especially if you run the lemon under hot water or warm it in the microwave for about 10 seconds.

Nutritional value
Per serving (1 piece)

Calories	133
Protein	4 g
Fat	6 g
Carbohydrate	15 g
Dietary Fiber	1 g
Calcium	51 mg

Percent of calories from

Protein	12%
Fat	43%
Carbohydrate	45%

● *Preheat oven to 400°F (200°C)*
● *Baking sheet, lined with parchment paper*

Filling

1	package (10.5 oz/290 g) silken firm tofu	1
2 tbsp	extra-virgin olive oil	25 mL
1	clove garlic, minced	1
1/4 cup	chopped green onions	50 mL
1/4 cup	chopped onion	50 mL
2	packages (each 10 oz/284 g) fresh spinach	2
1/4 cup	chopped fresh dill	50 mL
1/4 cup	chopped fresh parsley	50 mL
2 tbsp	freshly squeezed lemon juice	25 mL
1 tsp	salt	5 mL
1/4 tsp	freshly ground black pepper	1 mL
1	package (1 lb/500 g) strudel (phyllo) dough	1
1/3 cup	extra-virgin olive oil	75 mL
1 cup	soft fresh bread crumbs (see tip, opposite)	250 mL

1. *Prepare the filling:* Using a sieve, drain tofu.

2. In a large saucepan, heat oil over medium heat; cook garlic, green onions and onion until onions are softened, about 5 minutes. Transfer to a bowl and set aside.

3. Meanwhile, trim and rinse spinach, shaking off excess water. In the same saucepan, cook spinach, covered, until wilted. Uncover and continue cooking until moisture has evaporated. Add onion mixture, drained tofu, dill, parsley, lemon juice, salt and pepper; cook for a few minutes, until heated through, stirring to combine. Let cool.

4. Arrange 1 sheet of strudel dough on counter. Using a pastry brush, brush lightly with oil. Sprinkle with $1/3$ cup (75 mL) bread crumbs. Place second sheet of dough on top. Brush with oil and sprinkle with $1/3$ cup (75 mL) bread crumbs. Repeat once; top with sheet of dough to have 4 layers total.

5. Cut each sheet lengthwise into 4 strips. Place 2 tbsp (25 mL) filling at one corner and roll up to make a triangle. Repeat with remaining dough and filling to make about 24 pieces. Arrange on prepared baking sheet.

6. Bake in preheated oven for 20 to 25 minutes, or until golden brown.

TIP

A food processor or blender makes fresh bread crumbs in a flash, especially if you tear the bread into smaller pieces first. Two slices will make about 1 cup (250 mL) of crumbs. For added flavor and nutrition, use whole wheat bread.

MAKE AHEAD

Prepare through Step 5, cover with plastic wrap and foil and store in the freezer for up to 1 month. Bake frozen spanakopita in a preheated 375°F (190°C) oven for 25 to 35 minutes.

Kale Tart with Sun-Dried Tomatoes and Pine Nuts

Kale, that tangy relative to the cabbage, provides calcium to the diet. It can be found in the vegetable section of the supermarket. It looks very much like a large version of spinach, but it has a tougher texture that stands up well to boiling and sautéing to be at its delicious best.

MAKES 8 SERVINGS

TIP

Toast pine nuts on a baking sheet lined with parchment paper in a 350°F (180°C) oven for about 10 minutes, or just until fragrant. Don't be tempted to answer the telephone in the process — pine nuts burn easily, so watch them carefully!

Nutritional value
Per serving (1 piece)

Calories	339
Protein	10 g
Fat	21 g
Carbohydrate	28 g
Dietary Fiber	1 g
Calcium (a high source)	174 mg

Percent of calories from

Protein	11%
Fat	56%
Carbohydrate	33%

- Preheat oven to 425°F (220°C)
- 10-inch (25 cm) pie plate, ungreased

Pastry
1 1/2 cups	all-purpose flour	375 mL
3/4 tsp	salt	4 mL
1/2 cup	shortening	125 mL
1/4 cup	cold water	50 mL

Filling
1	package (10.25 oz/290 g) silken soft tofu	1
1 cup	water	250 mL
1	bunch (1 lb/500 g) kale	1
2 tbsp	extra-virgin olive oil	25 mL
2	cloves garlic, minced	2
2	eggs	2
1/3 cup	chopped drained sun-dried tomatoes packed in oil	75 mL
1 tsp	salt	5 mL
1/4 tsp	ground nutmeg	1 mL
1/4 tsp	freshly ground black pepper	1 mL
1/4 cup	toasted pine nuts (see tip, at left)	50 mL
1 tbsp	grated Parmesan cheese or crumbled extra-firm tofu	15 mL

1. *Prepare the pastry:* In a medium bowl, stir together flour and salt. Using a pastry blender, cut shortening into flour until mixture resembles fine crumbs. Stir in water all at once. Form pastry into a ball.

2. Roll out pastry between 2 sheets of waxed paper to fit pie plate. Remove top layer of waxed paper. Invert pie plate over pastry; invert plate. Discard waxed paper. Gently ease pastry into plate. Flute edges. Cover and refrigerate while you prepare the filling.

3. *Prepare the filling:* Using a sieve, drain tofu.

4. In a large saucepan, bring water to a boil and cook kale, covered, for 4 to 5 minutes, just until wilted. Drain and chop coarsely.

5. In the same saucepan, heat oil over medium heat. Cook garlic and chopped kale, stirring, for 2 to 3 minutes, or until tender. Remove from heat and set aside.

6. In a large bowl, whisk together drained tofu, eggs, sun-dried tomatoes, salt, nutmeg and pepper. Stir in kale mixture. Spoon into prepared pie shell. Sprinkle evenly with pine nuts and Parmesan cheese.

7. Bake in preheated oven until pastry is golden brown, about 20 minutes. Reduce heat to 350°F (180°C); bake for 25 to 30 minutes, or until filling is set. Serve warm or at room temperature.

TIP

Because pine nuts have a high fat content, they go rancid easily. To maintain their freshness, store them in a well-sealed plastic container in the freezer for up to 1 year.

MAKE AHEAD

Pastry shell may be covered and stored in the refrigerator for up to 1 day, or wrapped in plastic wrap, then in foil and stored in the freezer for up to 2 months.

Mushroom Strudel

Serve piping hot with a salad for lunch or in smaller portions as an appetizer.

MAKES 2 STRUDELS, ABOUT 14 PIECES

TIPS

Because leeks are grown mounded in sand, they often have grit or sand between the layers. To clean the leek, slice it lengthwise almost to the root and let tap water run through the various layers, removing any sand or grit.

Clean mushrooms with a damp cloth. Do not immerse them in water — they soak up water like a sponge.

Nutritional value
Per serving (1 piece)

Calories	303
Protein	6 g
Fat	9 g
Carbohydrate	22 g
Dietary Fiber	1 g
Calcium	64 mg (a source)

Percent of calories from

Protein	8%
Fat	27%
Carbohydrate	28%

- Preheat oven to 400°F (200°C)
- Baking sheet, lined with parchment paper

Filling

2 tbsp	vegetable oil	25 mL
1	leek, chopped	1
1	clove garlic, minced	1
12 oz	mushrooms, sliced	375 g
2 tbsp	freshly squeezed lemon juice	25 mL
2 tbsp	dry sherry (optional)	25 mL
1 tsp	dried thyme	5 mL
1 tsp	Worcestershire sauce	5 mL
1 tsp	salt	5 mL
½ tsp	ground nutmeg	2 mL
½ tsp	freshly ground black pepper	2 mL
12 oz	extra-firm tofu, crumbled	375 g
2 cups	fresh brown bread crumbs (about 4 slices)	500 mL
¼ cup	unblanched almonds	50 mL
¼ cup	chopped fresh parsley	50 mL
½	package (1 lb/500 g) strudel (phyllo) dough	½
¼ cup	vegetable oil	50 mL

1. *Prepare the filling:* In a Dutch oven or saucepan, heat oil over medium heat. Cook leek and garlic, covered, until leek is softened, about 5 minutes. Stir in mushrooms and cook, covered, until juices are released, about 5 minutes. Stir in lemon juice, sherry (if using), thyme, Worcestershire sauce, salt, nutmeg and pepper; cook, uncovered, until liquid is evaporated. Stir in tofu, bread crumbs, almonds and parsley; cook, stirring, for 2 minutes.

2. Arrange 1 sheet of strudel dough on counter. Using a pastry brush, brush lightly with oil. Place second sheet of dough on top; brush with oil. Repeat once; top with sheet of dough to have 4 layers total. Spread half of the mushroom mixture along long edge of dough. Roll up jelly-roll style. Repeat with 4 more sheets of dough and remaining filling.

3. Place on prepared baking sheet. Slice strudels almost all the way through on the diagonal into 2 inch (5 cm) thick pieces. Bake in preheated oven for 20 to 25 minutes, or until golden brown.

TIPS

For a stronger mushroom flavor, substitute portobello mushrooms for button mushrooms.

Remaining phyllo dough can be wrapped in plastic and frozen.

MAKE AHEAD

Cover and store in the refrigerator for up to 1 day, or wrap in plastic wrap, then in foil, and store in the freezer for up to 2 months.

Cocktail Crunch

Almonds and sesame seeds give this sophisticated nibble a calcium crunch with no lactose!

TIP

Unblanched almonds have their skins on and appear brown. Blanched almonds, without skins, are white. Unblanched almonds maintain freshness better than blanched almonds.

MAKE AHEAD

Place in a cookie tin and store at room temperature for up to 1 week.

Nutritional value
Per serving (¼ cup/50 mL)

Calories	109
Protein	3 g
Fat	8 g
Carbohydrate	9 g
Dietary Fiber (a source)	2 g
Calcium	26 mg

Percent of calories from

Protein	10%
Fat	60%
Carbohydrate	30%

- Preheat oven to 350°F (180°C)
- Baking sheet, lined with parchment paper

2 cups	mini shredded wheat squares	500 mL
2 cups	oat cereal rounds	500 mL
1 cup	pretzels (broken in half)	250 mL
1 cup	unblanched almonds	250 mL
¼ cup	sesame seeds	50 mL
½ tsp	salt	2 mL
½ tsp	dried basil	2 mL
½ tsp	dried rosemary	2 mL
¼ cup	vegetable oil	50 mL
1	clove garlic, minced	1
1 tbsp	Worcestershire sauce	15 mL

1. In a large bowl, combine shredded wheat squares, oat cereal rounds, pretzels, almonds, sesame seeds, salt, basil and rosemary.

2. In a small skillet, heat oil over medium heat. Stir-fry garlic until fragrant, about 30 seconds. Remove from heat.

3. Add oil, garlic and Worcestershire sauce to cereal mixture and toss to coat. Arrange in a single layer on prepared baking sheet.

4. Bake in preheated oven, stirring occasionally with a spoon, for 10 to 15 minutes, or until fragrant and pale brown. (Watch carefully, the mixture burns easily!) Let cool on a wire rack.

Salted Almonds

This calcium-bearing nibble is not too heavy to spoil appetites but is just right to titillate the palate when served with drinks before dinner. For added spice, try tossing with a little curry powder.

MAKES ABOUT 3 CUPS (750 ML)

MAKE AHEAD

Store in an airtight container at room temperature for up to 1 week or in the freezer for up to 2 months.

● *Preheat oven to 350°F (180°C)*
● *Baking sheet*

1 lb	unblanched almonds	500 g
2 tbsp	vegetable oil	25 mL
1 tsp	salt	5 mL

1. In a medium bowl, toss almonds with oil until lightly coated. Spread on baking sheet.

2. Bake in preheated oven for 12 to 15 minutes or until fragrant and deep golden brown.

3. Return almonds to bowl; toss with salt. Let cool.

Nutritional value
Per serving (1/3 cup/75 mL)

Calories	285
Protein	12 g
Fat	25 g
Carbohydrate	9 g
Dietary Fiber (a very high source)	7 g
Calcium (a high source)	178 mg

Percent of calories from

Protein	16%
Fat	73%
Carbohydrate	11%

Dried Fruit with Goat Cheese

Dried fruits such as figs, dates and apricots are all calcium sources, as are almonds. These delicious appetizers are perfect for lactose-intolerant people looking for alternative sources of calcium. For many, goat cheese (or chèvre) is well tolerated.

MAKES 24 APPETIZERS

TIP

If dried figs, apricots or dates seem dry and hard, simply pour boiling water over them, let them stand for 5 minutes, drain and pat dry with a paper towel.

MAKE AHEAD

Cover with plastic wrap and store in the refrigerator for up to 12 hours.

½ cup	mild soft chèvre cheese	125 mL
12	plump dried figs, halved, or pitted dates or dried apricots	12
12	unblanched almonds	12

1. Spread about 1 tsp (5 mL) chèvre in the center of the soft, cut side of each fig (or press into the center of each date or apricot). Press an almond into the center of the cheese. Arrange in concentric circles on an attractive platter.

Variation

Use a mixture of dried dates, apricots and figs.

Nutritional value
Per serving (2 appetizers)

Calories	116
Protein	3 g
Fat	4 g
Carbohydrate	18 g
Dietary Fiber (a high source)	4 g
Calcium	51 mg

Percent of calories from

Protein	11%
Fat	31%
Carbohydrate	58%

Breakfast, Brunch and Lunch

*M*any North Americans start the day with a bowl of cereal with milk. For lactose-intolerant people, cereal must be made without lactose (read the label, see page 13) and milk should be lactose-free or fortified soy milk. Here are some recipes using lactose-free milk, juices, stock, soy milk and tofu so you can begin your day free of symptoms.

Orange French Toast 52

French Toastwich 54

Apple French Toastwich 55

Make-Ahead Scramble 56

Potato Tortilla 58

Dilled Salmon Soufflé 60

Orange Pancakes 61

Basic Crêpes 62

Yeast Blini 63

Frittata 64

Basic Quiche 66

Orange French Toast

The best part of this vibrant way to start the day is that you can prepare it the night before. The hint of liqueur raises an ordinary recipe to the sublime.

TIPS

This lazy person's French toast is made even easier if you use a rasp to grate the orange zest. Rasps are available at cookware stores and have very sharp edges ideal for grating zest, Parmesan cheese and fresh nutmeg.

If bread is already sliced thinly, use two slices stacked on top of each other.

Nutritional Value
Per serving

Calories	377
Protein	12 g
Fat	7 g
Carbohydrate	65 g
Dietary Fiber (a source)	3 g
Calcium (a source)	105 mg

Percent of calories from

Protein	13%
Fat	17%
Carbohydrate	68%

● 13- by 9-inch (3 L) baking dish, greased

6	eggs	6
2 tbsp	grated orange zest	25 mL
1 cup	fortified orange juice	250 mL
2 tbsp	granulated sugar	25 mL
1 tbsp	orange-flavored liqueur (optional)	15 mL
1 tsp	vanilla	5 mL
6	slices (1 inch/2.5 cm thick) French bread	6

Orange Marmalade Sauce

1/2 cup	orange marmalade	125 mL
1/4 cup	fortified orange juice	50 mL
2 tbsp	liquid honey	25 mL
1 tbsp	orange-flavored liqueur (optional)	15 mL

1. In a medium bowl, beat together eggs, orange zest and juice, sugar, orange-flavored liqueur (if using) and vanilla.

2. Arrange bread, cutting to fit, in single layer in prepared baking dish. Pour orange mixture over top; cover and refrigerate overnight.

3. Preheat oven to 350°F (180°C). Bake, uncovered, for 25 to 30 minutes, or until no longer soggy and firm to the touch.

4. *Prepare the Orange Marmalade Sauce:* Meanwhile, in a small saucepan, bring marmalade, orange juice, honey and orange-flavored liqueur (if using) to a boil over high heat; reduce heat to medium and simmer, stirring, for about 5 minutes or until slightly thickened. Serve with French toast.

TIP

One medium orange will yield about 1 1/2 tbsp (22 mL) zest, so you'll likely need two for this recipe. Although I recommend using fortified orange juice in this recipe for added calcium, don't waste the flesh of the oranges after you zest them. Orange slices would taste terrific as a garnish for this dish.

French Toastwich

Make this no-fuss dish to eat with a salad and your favorite pickle for a sure-to-please lunch or supper.

MAKES 1 SERVING

2	slices bread	2
1 tsp	Dijon mustard	5 mL
1 tsp	light mayonnaise	5 mL
1 oz	shaved Black Forest ham, smoked turkey or smoked chicken	30 g
1	egg	1

1. Spread 1 slice of bread with mustard; spread remaining slice with mayonnaise. Sandwich ham between bread.

2. In a small bowl, whisk together egg and 1 tbsp (15 mL) water. Dip sandwich into mixture, turning to coat other side. Let stand for a few minutes until all liquid is absorbed.

3. Heat a nonstick skillet over medium-high heat; cook sandwich on both sides until golden brown and firm to the touch. Cut in half and serve at once.

Nutritional Value
Per serving

Calories	375
Protein	20 g
Fat	13 g
Carbohydrate	42 g
Dietary Fiber (a source)	2 g
Calcium (a source)	85 mg

Percent of calories from

Protein	22%
Fat	32%
Carbohydrate	46%

Apple French Toastwich

A variation on an old theme, this version is tasty with a dab of honey-mustard or fruit chutney. It doubles for breakfast or a light supper.

MAKES 1 SERVING

TIP

To make a strata: A strata is basically baked French toast. Try making your favorite sandwich, such as salmon salad, then pour beaten egg and water, lactose-free milk or soy milk over sandwich. Cover and refrigerate overnight. The next day, cook in a heated skillet or bake in a 350°F (180°C) oven for 40 to 45 minutes, or until puffed and firm to the touch.

2	slices raisin bread	2
1 tsp	Dijon mustard	5 mL
1 tsp	mayonnaise	5 mL
1 oz	shaved Black Forest ham, smoked turkey or smoked chicken	30 g
¼	apple, peeled, sliced and cored	¼
1	egg	1

1. Spread 1 slice of bread with mustard; spread remaining slice with mayonnaise. Sandwich ham and apple between bread.

2. In mixing bowl, whisk together egg and 1 tbsp (15 mL) water. Dip sandwich into mixture, turning to coat each side. Let stand for a few minutes until all liquid is absorbed.

3. Heat a nonstick skillet over medium-high heat; cook sandwich on both sides until golden brown and firm to the touch. Cut in half and serve at once.

Nutritional Value
Per serving

Calories	316
Protein	18 g
Fat	13 g
Carbohydrate	33 g
Dietary Fiber (a source)	2 g
Calcium (a source)	82 mg

Percent of calories from

Protein	22%
Fat	36%
Carbohydrate	42%

Make-Ahead Scramble

This is a variation of a popular egg casserole that I like to make for brunch because I can assemble it the night before. In the original, the cheese sauce helps keep the eggs moist for advance preparation. In this recipe, a tofu cream sauce and flavorful olive oil do the duty of cheese sauce with no lactose, less fat and lots of taste!

MAKES 4 SERVINGS

TIPS

Clean mushrooms with a damp cloth. Do not immerse them in water — they soak up water like a sponge.

Store fresh mushrooms in the refrigerator for up to 1 week in a paper bag rather than in plastic, where they are too moist and become slimy.

Nutritional Value
Per serving

Calories	409
Protein	23 g
Fat	24 g
Carbohydrate	27 g
Dietary Fiber (a source)	3 g
Calcium (a high source)	214 mg

Percent of calories from

Protein	22%
Fat	52%
Carbohydrate	26%

● *10-inch (25 cm) pie plate, greased*

1 tbsp	extra-virgin olive oil	15 mL
4 oz	mushrooms, sliced	125 g
3	green onions, chopped	3
8	eggs, beaten	8

Tofu Cream Sauce

1	package (10.25 oz/290 g) silken soft tofu	1
2 tbsp	light mayonnaise	25 mL
1 tbsp	freshly squeezed lemon juice	15 mL
1 tbsp	freshly grated Parmesan cheese (optional, if tolerated)	15 mL
1/4 tsp	salt	1 mL
Pinch	freshly ground black pepper	Pinch
Pinch	ground nutmeg	Pinch

Herbed Crumb Topping

1 cup	dry bread crumbs (see tip, opposite)	250 mL
1/4 cup	chopped fresh parsley	50 mL
1 tbsp	extra-virgin olive oil	15 mL
1 tbsp	freshly grated Parmesan cheese (optional, if tolerated)	15 mL
1/4 tsp	dried thyme	1 mL

1. In a large skillet, heat oil over medium heat; cook mushrooms and green onions for 5 minutes, or until softened. Add eggs and cook, stirring, for 5 to 7 minutes, or until eggs are just set. Remove from heat.

2. *Prepare the Tofu Cream Sauce:* Using a sieve, drain tofu. In a small bowl or food processor, beat together drained tofu, mayonnaise, lemon juice, cheese (if using), salt, pepper and nutmeg until smooth. Stir into eggs until well combined. Spoon into prepared pie plate.

3. *Prepare the Herbed Crumb Topping:* In a small bowl, combine bread crumbs, parsley, oil, cheese (if using) and thyme; sprinkle over eggs. Cover with plastic wrap and refrigerate overnight.

4. Preheat oven to 350°F (180°C). Bake for 25 to 30 minutes, or until heated through. Serve immediately.

Variation

Add 4 oz (125 g) chopped smoked ham or salmon just before spooning into pie plate.

TIPS

If you prefer, buy whole nutmeg and grate it with a rasp (available at cookware stores). The taste of freshly grated nutmeg is far superior to that of packaged ground nutmeg. The rasp will also work well to grate the Parmesan cheese, not to mention the zest of citrus fruits.

To make dry bread crumbs, toast bread, let it cool, then process it to fine crumbs in a blender or processor. Three slices will make about 1 cup (250 ml) of crumbs.

Potato Tortilla

This simple dish takes you on a quick trip to Spain. Serve the tortilla with crusty bread, olives, sliced tomato salad and Rioja wine.

MAKES 4 SERVINGS

TIPS

If you don't want to get teary, try freezing onions for 20 minutes before slicing or chopping.

A food processor or blender makes fresh bread crumbs in a flash, especially if you tear the bread into smaller pieces first. Two slices will make about 1 cup (250 mL) of crumbs. For added flavor and nutrition, use whole wheat bread.

Nutritional Value
Per serving

Calories	483
Protein	15 g
Fat	16 g
Carbohydrate	70 g
Dietary Fiber (a high source)	5 g
Calcium (a source)	132 mg

Percent of calories from

Protein	13%
Fat	30%
Carbohydrate	57%

- Preheat oven to 350°F (180°C)
- 9-inch (23 cm) pie plate, greased

3	large potatoes, peeled and quartered	3
2 tbsp	extra-virgin olive oil	25 mL
1	onion, chopped	1
1	clove garlic, minced	1
3	eggs	3
1 cup	fresh bread crumbs (see tip, at left)	250 mL
½ cup	chicken stock (store-bought or see recipe, page 68)	125 mL
¼ cup	chopped fresh parsley	50 mL
½ tsp	salt	2 mL
¼ tsp	freshly ground black pepper	1 mL
¼ tsp	ground nutmeg	1 mL

Seasoned Bread Crumbs

1 cup	fresh bread crumbs	250 mL
¼ cup	chopped fresh parsley	50 mL
1 tbsp	extra-virgin olive oil	15 mL
1 tbsp	freshly grated Parmesan cheese (optional, if tolerated)	15 mL
¼ tsp	freshly ground black pepper	1 mL
¼ tsp	dried thyme	1 mL

1. In a steamer, over simmering water, cook potatoes for 15 to 20 minutes, or until just tender. Cool and cube.

2. In a skillet, heat oil over medium-high heat; cook onion and garlic, covered, for 5 minutes, or until soft.

3. In a medium bowl, whisk together eggs, bread crumbs, chicken stock, parsley, salt, pepper and nutmeg. Stir in cubed potatoes and onion mixture. Spoon into prepared pie plate.

4. *Prepare the Seasoned Bread Crumbs:* In a small bowl, toss together bread crumbs, parsley, oil, cheese (if using), pepper and thyme; sprinkle over potato mixture.

5. Bake in preheated oven for 40 to 45 minutes, or until set. Let stand for 15 minutes before cutting into wedges. Serve hot or at room temperature.

MAKE AHEAD

Cover and store in the refrigerator for up to 1 day. Reheat, covered, in a preheated 350°F (180°C) oven for 20 to 25 minutes, or until warmed through.

Dilled Salmon Soufflé

If you want a simple recipe with a touch of glamour, try this soufflé. You can use sockeye or the less expensive pink salmon if you prefer. Remember to crush and include the bones for added calcium. Serve with crusty bread and a green salad for a quick but tasty treat.

MAKES 4 SERVINGS

TIPS

To judge whether egg whites are stiff enough once beaten, turn the bowl almost upside down. If whites stay intact and inside, they are stiff.

Leftover egg yolks can be covered and refrigerated for a day. Mixed with a spoonful of water, they can be painted on breads, cookies and pastry to give a golden sheen. They can be saved to make scrambled eggs or used to make a custard.

Nutritional Value
Per serving

Calories	303
Protein	22 g
Fat	14 g
Carbohydrate	21 g
Dietary Fiber	1 g
Calcium (a high source)	215 mg

Percent of calories from

Protein	29%
Fat	43%
Carbohydrate	27%

- Preheat oven to 400°F (200°C)
- 6-cup (1.5 L) soufflé dish or straight-sided baking dish, ungreased

1	can (7.5 oz/213 g) salmon	1
6	eggs, separated	6
1 cup	fresh bread crumbs	250 mL
2 tbsp	freshly squeezed lemon juice	25 mL
2 tbsp	chopped fresh dill	25 mL
1 tsp	Worcestershire sauce	5 mL
½ tsp	salt	2 mL
½ tsp	dry mustard	2 mL
Pinch	cayenne pepper	Pinch

1. Drain salmon; discard skin and mash bones.

2. In a medium bowl, beat together salmon with mashed bones, 5 egg yolks, bread crumbs, lemon juice, dill, Worcestershire sauce, salt, mustard and cayenne pepper until well combined. Set aside.

3. In a separate bowl, using clean beaters, beat egg whites on high speed until stiff peaks form. Fold about one-third into salmon mixture to lighten. Gently fold in remaining egg whites.

4. Spoon into soufflé dish. Bake in preheated oven for 25 to 30 minutes, or until soufflé is set but center is still slightly moist. Serve immediately.

Orange Pancakes

The secret to these tender pancakes is cake-and-pastry flour. They may be served with the usual maple syrup or spread with marmalade. You won't miss butter. To make a mini sandwich, use a tablespoon (15 mL) of batter to make each pancake and spread with marmalade. It's the perfect size for a child's breakfast or snack.

MAKES ABOUT TWELVE 4-INCH/10 CM PANCAKES

MAKE AHEAD

Stack pancakes separated with waxed paper, double-wrap stack in foil and store in the refrigerator for up to 2 days or in the freezer for up to 3 months. Defrost in the refrigerator overnight and reheat in the microwave or toaster.

2 cups	cake-and-pastry flour	500 mL
1/4 cup	granulated sugar	50 mL
2 tsp	baking powder	10 mL
1/2 tsp	baking soda	2 mL
1/2 tsp	salt	2 mL
1	egg	1
1 cup	fortified orange juice	250 mL
3 tbsp	vegetable oil	45 mL

1. In a medium bowl, sift together flour, sugar, baking powder, baking soda and salt.

2. In a measuring cup, whisk together egg, orange juice and oil. Pour into dry ingredients, stirring with a fork just until dry ingredients are moistened.

3. Heat a nonstick skillet over medium-high heat. For each pancake, spoon 1/4 cup (50 mL) batter into pan. Cook until bubbles appear and break. Flip and cook until second side is golden brown. Serve at once.

Nutritional Value
Per serving (1 pancake)

Calories	125
Protein	2 g
Fat	4 g
Carbohydrate	20 g
Dietary Fiber	1 g
Calcium	8 mg

Percent of calories from

Protein	7%
Fat	29%
Carbohydrate	64%

Basic Crêpes

*Somehow crêpes always seem special. They can be filled with a sweet or savory filling —
a great way to use up leftovers. It's worth making a batch and keeping some in the freezer
for emergencies. Just wrap in plastic wrap, separating each crêpe with a piece of waxed
paper and double-wrapping in foil to protect them from freezer burn. They will keep
frozen for up to 3 months.*

**MAKES 10 TO 16 CRÊPES
OR ABOUT 30 MINI CRÊPES**

MAKE AHEAD

Cover and store in the
refrigerator for up to
1 day.

1 cup	all-purpose flour	250 mL
1 tsp	granulated sugar	5 mL
½ tsp	salt	2 mL
2	eggs	2
1½ cups	lactose-free milk or fortified soy milk	375 mL
1 tbsp	vegetable oil	15 mL

1. In a small bowl, stir together flour, sugar and salt.

2. In a measuring cup, whisk together eggs, milk and oil;
pour into dry ingredients and whisk until smooth.
Cover and refrigerate for at least 1 hour or overnight.

3. Spray a nonstick skillet with nonstick baking spray
and heat over medium-high heat. For each crêpe, spoon
2 tbsp (25 mL) batter into pan for a 5-inch (12 cm)
appetizer-size crêpe or ¼ cup (50 mL) for a dessert-
or dinner-size crêpe, tilting pan to coat bottom. Cook
until pale brown around edges and starting to pull away
from pan. Flip and cook until second side is browned.

4. Stack crêpes on a plate, separating with pieces of
waxed paper.

Nutritional Value
Per serving (1 of 10 crêpes)

Calories	92
Protein	4 g
Fat	3 g
Carbohydrate	12 g
Dietary Fiber	0 g
Calcium	52 mg

Percent of calories from

Protein	16%
Fat	32%
Carbohydrate	52%

For a savory hors d'oeuvre, spoon a dab of your favorite
sandwich filling (salmon, tuna) onto mini crêpes and
garnish with chopped green onions or dill sprigs.

For a delicious main course, fill the large crêpes with
creamy mushroom and chicken filling (see Chicken Pot
Pie recipe, page 134) and roll up.

For a quick dessert idea, squeeze lemon juice over large
crêpes, sprinkle with granulated sugar and fold into
quarters. Serve with sliced fresh strawberries, blueberries
or raspberries.

Yeast Blini

These savory pancakes may be served at breakfast, lunch or dinner. Make mini blini and serve with yogurt, if tolerated, and caviar or smoked salmon as an appetizer. Or make them full-size and serve with Quick Strawberry Sauce or the blueberry variation (see recipe, page 259).

MAKES ABOUT SIXTEEN 4-INCH/10 CM BLINI OR ABOUT 30 MINI BLINI

1/2 cup	lukewarm water	125 mL
1 tbsp	active dry yeast (one 1/4 oz/7 g package)	15 mL
2 tsp	granulated sugar	10 mL
2	eggs, beaten	2
1 cup	all-purpose flour	250 mL
3/4 cup	lukewarm beer, lactose-free milk or fortified soy milk	175 mL
1/2 cup	whole wheat flour	125 mL
2 tbsp	vegetable oil	25 mL
1/2 tsp	salt	2 mL

1. Rinse a large bowl with hot water; dry well. Pour in lukewarm water; sprinkle yeast and sugar over water. Let stand in a warm place for 10 minutes or until yeast is foamy.

2. Gradually whisk in eggs, all-purpose flour, beer, whole wheat flour, oil and salt until smooth.

3. Cover bowl with plastic wrap and set in a pan of warm water until batter has doubled in size, about 1 hour. Stir down batter.

4. Heat a nonstick skillet over medium-high heat. For each blini, spoon into skillet 1 tbsp (15 mL) batter for mini size or 1/4 cup (50 mL) batter for larger size; cook for about 1 minute, or until bubbles break on top and underside is golden brown. Flip and cook until second side is golden brown.

Nutritional Value
Per serving (1/16th of recipe)

Calories	71
Protein	2 g
Fat	2 g
Carbohydrate	10 g
Dietary Fiber	1 g
Calcium	7 mg

Percent of calories from

Protein	13%
Fat	28%
Carbohydrate	55%

Frittata

This oven-baked version is a cinch to make and can be rich in calcium, depending on the ingredients chosen.

TIPS

A frittata is an Italian omelet that is traditionally cooked in a heavy frying pan, then finished off under the broiler. In this simpler version, you just combine the ingredients, then bake the frittata in a pie plate.

Use a blender or food processor to make fresh bread crumbs from sliced bread. For this recipe, you'll need about 1 slice of bread.

Nutritional Value
Per serving (¼th of recipe)

Calories	227
Protein	12 g
Fat	13 g
Carbohydrate	16 g
Dietary Fiber (a source)	3 g
Calcium (a high source)	208 mg

Percent of calories from

Protein	21%
Fat	51%
Carbohydrate	27%

● *Preheat oven to 350°F (180°C)*
● *9-inch (23 cm) pie plate*

½ cup	fresh bread crumbs (see tip, at left)	125 mL
1	bunch broccoli, broken into florets and steamed	1
½	red bell pepper, sliced	½
2 tbsp	vegetable oil	25 mL
1	onion, chopped	1
½ tsp	dried thyme	2 mL
¾ cup	shredded old Cheddar cheese (optional, if tolerated)	175 mL
4	eggs	4
¼ cup	lactose-free milk or fortified soy milk	50 mL
½ tsp	salt	2 mL
¼ tsp	ground nutmeg	1 mL
¼ tsp	freshly ground black pepper	1 mL

1. Using blender or food processor, make bread crumbs. Sprinkle bread crumbs over bottom of pie plate.

2. Arrange broccoli and red pepper evenly over bread crumbs.

3. In a small skillet, heat oil over medium-high heat; cook onion, covered, until softened, about 5 minutes. Stir in thyme. Sprinkle onion mixture and cheese (if using) over broccoli and peppers.

4. In a small bowl, whisk together eggs, milk, salt, nutmeg and pepper. Pour over vegetables.

5. Bake in preheated oven for 35 to 40 minutes, or until puffed and golden brown. Let cool on a wire rack for at least 15 minutes before slicing, or serve at room temperature.

Variation

Substitute 3 cups (750 mL) of another calcium-rich vegetable, such as blanched kale, bok choy or napa cabbage, for the broccoli.

TIP

Some lactose-intolerant people can handle small quantities of hard aged cheeses such as old Cheddar and Parmesan without a problem. Whether to include cheese must be considered on an individual basis.

Basic Quiche

One of the most versatile recipes, quiche can be served for breakfast, lunch or supper. Here's one for the lactose intolerant.

MAKES 6 SERVINGS

TIP

An ovenproof glass pie plate browns the pastry better than a shiny metal pan.

- Preheat oven to 425°F (220°C)
- 9-inch (23 cm) pie plate

1	unbaked 9-inch (23 cm) pie shell	1
4	strips side bacon, chopped and cooked	4
¾ cup	shredded old Cheddar cheese (optional, if tolerated)	175 mL
3	eggs	3
1 cup	lactose-free milk or fortified soy milk	250 mL
½ tsp	salt	2 mL
¼ tsp	ground nutmeg	1 mL
¼ tsp	freshly ground black pepper	1 mL

1. Press pie shell into pie plate. Sprinkle bacon and cheese (if using) over bottom of pie shell.

2. In a small bowl, whisk together eggs, milk, salt, nutmeg and pepper. Pour over cheese and bacon.

3. Bake in preheated oven for 10 minutes. Reduce heat to 350°F (180°C) and bake for 30 to 35 minutes, or until top is puffed and golden brown and pastry is brown. Let cool on a wire rack for at least 15 minutes before slicing, or serve at room temperature.

Variation

For a calcium-rich version with vitamin D, substitute 1 can (7.5 oz/213 g) salmon, drained and crumbled, with mashed bones, for the bacon. Sprinkle 1 tbsp (15 mL) chopped fresh dill over the salmon.

Nutritional Value	
Per serving	
Calories	286
Protein	11 g
Fat	21 g
Carbohydrate	13 g
Dietary Fiber	0 g
Calcium (a high source)	171 mg
Percent of calories from	
Protein	15%
Fat	67%
Carbohydrate	18%

Soups

There is a soup to please every palate and every lifestyle. In addition to your favorite vegetable, chunky meat or bean soups, you can continue to enjoy cream soups and chowders, which normally use milk, cream and butter. Vegetable oil, olive oil or a little water replaces butter to sauté vegetables. A vegetable purée thickens soup, giving it a smooth consistency with no lactose. When soups need to be thinned, use stock, lactose free milk, fortified soy milk or even fruit juice to create the desired consistency.

With vegetable purées and a minimum of vegetable oil for cooking, these soups have a lower fat level than the traditional recipes.

Happily, soups can fill the role of lunch or a simple supper when accompanied with good bread and a salad. Soups can be made ahead and, in most cases, frozen for up to 2 months. Simply pour into a plastic container such as a yogurt or margarine tub, label, and freeze. They can be reheated directly from frozen, making them ideal to tote along for a work lunch, providing a microwave oven or stove is available. If not, simply reheat and fill a Thermos.

Basic Chicken Stock 68
Turkey Stock 69
Chicken Tofu Noodle Soup 70
Broccoli Tarragon Soup 71
Minestrone 72
Curried Parsnip Soup 74
French Onion Soup 75

Leek and Potato Soup 76
Sweet Potato–Orange Soup 77
Creamy Pumpkin and Apple Soup . . . 78
Cream of Carrot Soup 79
Mushroom Chowder 80
Salmon Chowder 81
Creamy Clam Chowder 82

Basic Chicken Stock

Nothing beats the flavor added to soups and stews from the taste of homemade chicken stock. As a bonus, the stock contains some calcium leached from the bones during the cooking process.

MAKES ABOUT 15 CUPS (3.75 L)

TIPS

Be sure to date and label all your containers so you can use up the oldest first.

If you're not planning to use the stock right away, you can leave the fat on to act as a seal; discard it before you use the stock.

MAKE AHEAD

Store in the refrigerator for up to 3 days or in the freezer for up to 4 months.

Nutritional value
Per serving (1 cup/250 mL)

Calories	271
Protein	21 g
Fat	19 g
Carbohydrate	2 g
Dietary Fiber	1 g
Calcium	39 mg

Percent of calories from

Protein	32%
Fat	65%
Carbohydrate	3%

3½ lbs	chicken necks or backs	1.75 kg
3	sprigs fresh parsley	3
2	bay leaves	2
1	carrot, peeled and coarsely chopped	1
1	stalk celery, coarsely chopped	1
1	onion, stuck with 6 whole cloves and halved	1
2 tbsp	freshly squeezed lemon juice	25 mL
1 tsp	black peppercorns	5 mL
1 tsp	dried thyme	5 mL
	Salt and freshly ground black pepper	

1. Rinse chicken necks and place in a 26-cup (6.5 L) saucepan or stockpot. Add parsley, bay leaves, carrot, celery, onion halves stuck with cloves, lemon juice, peppercorns and thyme. Add enough cold water to cover. Bring to a boil over high heat, skimming off any foam that rises. Reduce heat to low and simmer, uncovered, for 1½ hours. Remove from heat.

2. Set a fine-mesh sieve over a large bowl. Ladle stock through sieve into bowl, leaving behind dregs. Discard vegetables and herbs. Strip any chicken meat from bones and reserve for another use. Season stock to taste with salt and pepper.

3. If not using stock immediately, pour into 2-cup (500 mL) and 4-cup (1 L) airtight containers. Cover and refrigerate for 1 to 2 hours, until chilled. Skim off any fat and discard.

Variation

Turkey backs or necks can be substituted for the chicken pieces.

Turkey Stock

Don't throw out that turkey carcass! You have the makings of a great soup, bursting with flavor and calcium from those bones. If you don't feel like making it now, simply freeze the carcass in a freezer bag until you can transform it into a hearty soup or casserole.

TIP

Plastic yogurt and sour cream containers are ideal for freezing stock.

MAKE AHEAD

Store in the refrigerator for up to 3 days or in the freezer for up to 4 months.

1	turkey carcass, broken into pieces	1
6	whole peppercorns	6
4	sprigs fresh parsley	4
2	carrots, peeled and chopped	2
2	stalks celery, chopped	2
1	onion, studded with 6 whole cloves	1
1	bay leaf	1
2 tbsp	freshly squeezed lemon juice	25 mL
1 tsp	dried thyme	5 mL

1. Place turkey carcass pieces in a large saucepan or stockpot. Add peppercorns, parsley, carrots, celery, onion stuck with whole cloves, bay leaf, lemon juice and thyme. Add enough cold water to cover. Bring to a boil over high heat, skimming off any foam that rises. Reduce heat to low and simmer, uncovered, for $1\frac{1}{2}$ hours. Remove from heat and let cool.

2. Skim off any fat and discard. Set a fine-mesh sieve over a large bowl. Ladle stock through sieve into bowl, leaving behind dregs. Discard vegetables and herbs. Strip turkey meat from carcass and reserve for soup.

3. If not using stock immediately, pour into 2-cup (500 mL) and 4-cup (1 L) airtight containers and let cool. Date and label containers.

Nutritional value
Per serving (1 cup/250 mL)

Calories	289
Protein	31 g
Fat	16 g
Carbohydrate	3 g
Dietary Fiber	1 g
Calcium	53 mg

Percent of calories from

Protein	43%
Fat	52%
Carbohydrate	5%

Chicken Tofu Noodle Soup

Considered a cure for everything from a cold to a bad day, this soothing soup can be made in minutes with ready-made chicken stock.

MAKES ABOUT 8 CUPS (2 L)

TIPS

If you do not have any cooked chicken, substitute one 6-oz (175 g) chopped chicken breast.

For an extra boost of calcium, choose tofu made with calcium chloride or calcium sulfate.

MAKE AHEAD

Ladle into an airtight container and store in the refrigerator for up to 2 days.

Nutritional value
Per serving (1 cup/250 mL)

Calories	183
Protein	11 g
Fat	7 g
Carbohydrate	19 g
Dietary Fiber	1 g
Calcium (a source)	90 mg

Percent of calories from

Protein	24%
Fat	36%
Carbohydrate	41%

2 tbsp	vegetable oil	25 mL
1	leek (white and light green parts only), thinly sliced	1
1	bay leaf	1
8 oz	firm tofu, diced	250 g
4 oz	tiny pasta or thin noodles	125 g
6 cups	Basic Chicken Stock (see recipe, page 68)	1.5 L
1 cup	diced cooked chicken	250 mL
1 tsp	salt	5 mL
1/4 tsp	freshly ground black pepper	1 mL
1/4 cup	chopped fresh parsley	50 mL

1. In a large saucepan, heat oil over medium heat. Stir-fry leek until softened, about 2 minutes. Add bay leaf, tofu, pasta, chicken stock, chicken, salt and pepper; increase heat to high and bring to a boil. Reduce heat to low and simmer, uncovered, for about 20 minutes to allow flavors to blend. Stir in parsley.

Variations

Use cooked turkey and turkey stock (see recipe, page 69).

Add 1 to 2 cups (250 to 500 mL) calcium vegetables, such as bok choy or kale.

Broccoli Tarragon Soup

Broccoli is a vegetable source of calcium. As well, the calcium content of the soup can be enriched by garnishing with a spoonful of yogurt, providing yogurt is tolerated. Otherwise, serve with Yogurt Substitute or Sour Cream Substitute (see recipes, below).

MAKES ABOUT 5 CUPS (1.25 L)

MAKE AHEAD

Ladle into an airtight container and store in the refrigerator for up to 2 days or in the freezer for up to 2 months.

1	bunch broccoli	1
1	onion, chopped	1
1	potato, peeled and chopped	1
1	bay leaf	1
3 cups	Basic Chicken Stock (see recipe, page 68)	750 mL
1 tbsp	dried tarragon	15 mL
	Salt and freshly ground black pepper	
¼ cup	plain yogurt (if tolerated), Yogurt Substitute or Sour Cream Substitute (see recipes, below)	50 mL

1. Trim tough parts of broccoli stem. Coarsely chop broccoli.

2. In a large saucepan, combine broccoli, onion, potato, bay leaf, chicken stock and tarragon. Bring to a boil over high heat; reduce heat to medium, cover and simmer for 20 to 25 minutes, or until vegetables are tender. Discard bay leaf.

3. In a blender or food processor, puree soup in batches. Season to taste with salt and pepper.

4. Ladle into serving bowls and garnish each with a dollop of yogurt.

Yogurt Substitute

In a small bowl, stir together 1 cup (250 mL) drained silken soft tofu with 1 tbsp (15 mL) vegetable oil and 1 tbsp (15 mL) freshly squeezed lemon juice until smooth. Makes about 1 cup (250 mL).

Sour Cream Substitute

In a small bowl, stir together 1 cup (250 mL) drained soft tofu with 1 tbsp (15 mL) light mayonnaise and 1 tbsp (15 mL) freshly squeezed lemon juice until smooth. Makes about 1 cup (250 mL).

Nutritional value
Per serving (1 cup/250 mL)

Calories	105
Protein	8 g
Fat	1 g
Carbohydrate	18 g
Dietary Fiber (a source)	3 g
Calcium (a source)	88 mg

Percent of calories from

Protein	27%
Fat	11%
Carbohydrate	63%

Minestrone

This hearty soup contains calcium from three sources: kale, chicken stock and beans.
Serve with Tortilla Chips (see recipe, page 35) or sesame bread for an added boost of calcium.

**MAKES ABOUT 9 CUPS
(2.25 L)**

TIPS

For convenience, use canned soybeans, available in some supermarkets or health food stores, instead of dried beans. All beans contain some calcium, but soybeans contain the most.

Some lactose-intolerant people can tolerate hard aged cheeses such as Parmesan, while others cannot. This is an individual matter and must be judged accordingly.

Nutritional value
Per serving (1 cup/250 mL)

Calories	179
Protein	11 g
Fat	8 g
Carbohydrate	20 g
Dietary Fiber (a high source)	4 g
Calcium (a source)	147 mg

Percent of calories from

Protein	23%
Fat	36%
Carbohydrate	41%

2 tbsp	olive oil	25 mL
1	large onion, chopped	1
2	carrots, chopped	2
2	stalks celery, chopped	2
1	clove garlic, minced	1
1	can (28 oz/796 mL) chopped tomatoes	1
1	can (19 oz/540 mL) soybeans, drained and rinsed	1
4 cups	coarsely chopped kale leaves, stems removed	1 L
3 cups	Basic Chicken Stock (see recipe, page 68) or Turkey Stock (see recipe, page 69)	750 mL
1 tsp	dried basil	5 mL
1/2 tsp	dried oregano	2 mL
1	bay leaf	1
1/2 tsp	salt	2 mL
1/4 tsp	freshly ground black pepper	1 mL
Dash	hot pepper sauce	Dash
	Freshly grated Parmesan cheese (optional, if tolerated)	

1. In a large saucepan or Dutch oven, heat oil over medium heat. Cook onion, covered, until softened, about 5 minutes. Stir in carrots, celery and garlic; cook for 5 minutes, until softened. If mixture seems dry, stir in about 1/2 cup (125 mL) water or stock to prevent scorching.

2. Stir in tomatoes with juice, soybeans, kale, stock, basil, oregano, bay leaf, salt, pepper and hot pepper sauce. Reduce heat to low and simmer, uncovered, for 20 to 25 minutes, to allow flavors to blend. Taste and adjust seasoning as desired with hot sauce, salt and pepper. Discard bay leaf.

3. Ladle into serving bowls and sprinkle with Parmesan cheese, if tolerated.

Variation

If you prefer, substitute canned navy beans or chickpeas for soybeans.

MAKE AHEAD

Prepare through Step 2, ladle into an airtight container and store in the refrigerator for up to 3 days or in the freezer for up to 3 months.

Curried Parsnip Soup

Served hot or cold, this soup has a nutty, sweet flavor that is complemented by a crunchy calcium topping of toasted almonds.

MAKES ABOUT 8 CUPS (2 L)

TIP

Toasting nuts intensifies their flavor. To toast almonds, bake in preheated 350°F (180°C) oven for 10 to 12 minutes, or until golden brown and fragrant.

MAKE AHEAD

Ladle into an airtight container and store in the refrigerator for up to 2 days or in the freezer for up to 2 months.

Nutritional value
Per serving (1 cup/250 mL)

Calories	170
Protein	7 g
Fat	4 g
Carbohydrate	30 g
Dietary Fiber (a very high source)	8 g
Calcium (a source)	73 mg

Percent of calories from

Protein	15%
Fat	18%
Carbohydrate	67%

● Baking sheet

1	onion, chopped	1
1	pear, peeled, cored and quartered	1
1	bay leaf	1
2 lbs	parsnips, peeled and chopped	1 kg
5 cups	Basic Chicken Stock (see recipe, page 68)	1.25 L
1 tsp	curry powder	5 mL
1 cup	fortified soy milk or 2% lactose-free milk	250 mL
½ tsp	salt	2 mL
¼ tsp	freshly ground black pepper	1 mL
¼ cup	toasted chopped unblanched almonds (see tip, at left)	50 mL

1. In a large saucepan, combine onion, pear, bay leaf, parsnips, chicken stock and curry powder. Bring to a boil over high heat; reduce heat to medium, cover and simmer for 25 to 30 minutes, or until parsnips are very tender. Discard bay leaf.

2. In a blender or food processor, purée soup in batches. Stir in milk, salt and pepper. Reheat gently in saucepan.

3. Ladle into serving bowls and garnish with almonds.

French Onion Soup

You will love this lactose-free version of a classic, ideal for a cozy supper on a blustery day. Serve with crusty bread, a salad and a glass of wine.

MAKES ABOUT 6 CUPS (1.5 L)

MAKE AHEAD

Prepare through Step 1, ladle into an airtight container and store in the refrigerator for up to 1 day.

● *8-cup (2 L) casserole dish or 6 ovenproof French onion soup bowls*

2 tbsp	vegetable oil	25 mL
5	large Vidalia or cooking onions, halved and thinly sliced	5
2 tbsp	all-purpose flour	25 mL
6 cups	Basic Chicken Stock (see recipe, page 68)	1.5 L
1	bay leaf	1
1/2 cup	dry white wine	125 mL
1/2 tsp	dried thyme	2 mL
1/4 tsp	freshly ground black pepper	1 mL
1	clove garlic, peeled and halved	1
6	slices French baguette	6
1/4 cup to 1/2 cup	freshly grated Parmesan cheese (optional, if tolerated)	50 to 125 mL

1. In a large saucepan, heat oil over medium-high heat. Cook onions, covered, for 25 to 30 minutes, or until very soft. Stir in flour. Gradually pour in chicken stock, stirring constantly to prevent lumps forming. Stir in bay leaf, white wine, thyme and pepper. Cook, uncovered, for 20 to 25 minutes, or until thickened. Taste and adjust seasoning as desired with thyme and pepper. Meanwhile, preheat the broiler.

2. Brush garlic clove against each slice of bread and sprinkle with cheese (if using).

3. Ladle soup into casserole dish or individual soup bowls; arrange bread slices on top. Place under broiler and broil for 30 to 60 seconds, or until toasts are golden brown. Serve immediately.

Nutritional value	
Per serving (1 cup/250 mL)	
Calories	329
Protein	13 g
Fat	11 g
Carbohydrate	42 g
Dietary Fiber (a source)	3 g
Calcium (a source)	157 mg
Percent of calories from	
Protein	16%
Fat	29%
Carbohydrate	51%

Leek and Potato Soup

A hearty soup for a blustery day, this soup is traditionally made with cream. My version gives the same rich sensation, but with no dairy product!

MAKES ABOUT 8 CUPS (2 L)

TIP

To minimize fat content, add a little water instead of more oil to help vegetables soften without scorching.

MAKE AHEAD

Ladle into an airtight container and store in the refrigerator for up to 2 days or in the freezer for up to 4 months.

1 tbsp	vegetable oil	25 mL
2	leeks (white and pale green parts only), cleaned and sliced	2
4	potatoes, peeled and diced (1 ¼ lbs/625 g)	4
1	bay leaf	1
4 cups	Basic Chicken Stock (see recipe, page 68)	1 L
½ tsp	dried thyme	2 mL
½ tsp	freshly ground black pepper	2 mL
	Salt	
	Whole Wheat Croutons (see recipe, page 251) or 2 green onions, chopped	

1. In a large saucepan, heat oil over medium heat. Cook leeks, covered, until softened, about 5 minutes. Add potatoes, bay leaf, chicken stock, thyme and pepper. Increase heat to high and bring to a boil; reduce heat to medium, cover and simmer until potatoes are very tender, about 20 minutes. Discard bay leaf. Taste and add salt if desired.

2. Ladle into serving bowls and garnish with croutons.

Leeks are grown in sand. As a result, you need to wash them thoroughly so the sand doesn't end up in the soup! Trim the root end and cut the leek to use only the white and pale green parts (the rest is too coarse.) Slice it lengthwise and rinse under cold running water to penetrate all the crevices and remove any sand.

Nutritional value
Per serving (1 cup/250 mL)

Calories	125
Protein	4 g
Fat	4 g
Carbohydrate	19 g
Dietary Fiber (a source)	2 g
Calcium	32 mg

Percent of calories from

Protein	13%
Fat	27%
Carbohydrate	60%

Sweet Potato–Orange Soup

Rich and oh-so-smooth, this soup is creamy without cream! Serve with homemade Whole Wheat Croutons (see recipe, page 251).

MAKES ABOUT 8 CUPS (2 L)

TIP

If you use a commercial chicken stock, keep in mind that they tend to be saltier than homemade stocks. Taste before adding salt.

MAKE AHEAD

Ladle into an airtight container and store in the refrigerator for up to 3 days or in the freezer for up to 2 months.

2 lbs	sweet potatoes, peeled and sliced (about 3 large)	1 kg
2 cups	Basic Chicken Stock (see recipe, page 68)	500 mL
2 cups	fortified orange juice	500 mL
1 cup	water	250 mL
1	onion, chopped	1
1	bay leaf	1
1 tsp	dried thyme	5 mL
½ cup	fortified soy milk or 2% lactose-free milk	125 mL
½ tsp	salt	2 mL
¼ tsp	freshly ground black pepper	1 mL

1. In a large saucepan, combine potatoes, chicken stock, orange juice, water, onion, bay leaf and thyme. Bring to a boil over high heat; reduce heat to medium, cover and simmer for 25 to 30 minutes, or until potatoes are very tender. Discard bay leaf.

2. In a blender or food processor, purée soup in batches. Add milk, salt and pepper; blend well. Gently reheat if necessary to serve.

Nutritional value
Per serving (1 cup/250 mL)

Calories	138
Protein	4 g
Fat	1 g
Carbohydrate	30 g
Dietary Fiber (a high source)	4 g
Calcium	41 mg

Percent of calories from

Protein	11%
Fat	5%
Carbohydrate	84%

Creamy Pumpkin and Apple Soup

Truly a harvest blend made from pumpkin and apple, this soup is puréed and has a velvety texture. For a calcium boost, serve with a spoonful of yogurt, if tolerated, or Yogurt Substitute (see box, page 71).

MAKES ABOUT 6 CUPS (1.5 L)

MAKE AHEAD

Ladle into an airtight container and store in the refrigerator for up to 2 days or in the freezer for up to 2 months.

2 tbsp	vegetable oil	25 mL
2	stalks celery, sliced (1 cup/250 mL)	2
1	large onion, chopped	1
1	can (14 oz/398 mL) pumpkin purée (not pie filling)	1
1	apple, peeled, cored and quartered	1
1	bay leaf	1
3 cups	Basic Chicken Stock (see recipe, page 68)	750 mL
1 tsp	curry powder	5 mL
¼ tsp	freshly ground black pepper	1 mL
	Salt	

1. In a large saucepan, heat oil over medium heat. Cook celery and onion, covered, until softened, about 5 minutes. Stir in pumpkin purée, apple, bay leaf, chicken stock and curry powder. Increase heat to high and bring to a boil; reduce heat to medium, cover and simmer until vegetables are tender, about 20 minutes. Discard bay leaf.

2. In a blender or food processor, purée soup in batches. Stir in pepper and salt to taste.

Nutritional value
Per serving (1 cup/250 mL)

Calories	101
Protein	4 g
Fat	5 g
Carbohydrate	12 g
Dietary Fiber (a source)	3 g
Calcium	43 mg

Percent of calories from

Protein	14%
Fat	41%
Carbohydrate	45%

Cream of Carrot Soup

A vibrant harvest soup, this is perfect served with a spoonful of yogurt, if tolerated, or Yogurt Substitute (see box, page 71) and a grating of fresh nutmeg. To save time, make the most of packaged frozen butternut squash!

MAKES ABOUT 6 CUPS (1.5 L)

TIP

This soup is quite thick. If you prefer a thinner soup, simply add more fortified soy milk or lactose-free milk.

MAKE AHEAD

Ladle into an airtight container and store in the refrigerator for up to 2 days or in the freezer for up to 2 months.

Nutritional value
Per serving (1 cup/250 mL)

Calories	123
Protein	5 g
Fat	5 g
Carbohydrate	17 g
Dietary Fiber (a high source)	4 g
Calcium (a source)	69 mg

Percent of calories from

Protein	14%
Fat	35%
Carbohydrate	51%

2 tbsp	vegetable oil	25 mL
1	onion, chopped	1
1	clove garlic, minced	1
1	bay leaf	1
5	large carrots (about 1 ½ lbs/750 g), peeled and chopped	5
3 cups	Basic Chicken Stock (see recipe, page 68)	750 mL
½ cup	fortified soy milk or 2% lactose-free milk	125 mL
½ tsp	salt	2 mL
½ tsp	ground nutmeg	2 mL
¼ tsp	freshly ground black pepper	1 mL

1. In a large saucepan, heat oil over medium heat. Cook onion and garlic, covered, until onion is softened, about 5 minutes. Add bay leaf, carrots and chicken stock. Increase heat to high and bring to a boil; reduce heat to medium, cover and simmer for 20 to 30 minutes, or until carrots are very tender. Discard bay leaf.

2. In a blender or food processor, purée soup in batches. Stir in milk, salt, nutmeg and pepper. Taste and add more salt if necessary.

Variation

Cream of Butternut Squash Soup: Substitute 4 cups (1 L) cubed peeled butternut squash (fresh or frozen) for the carrots.

Mushroom Chowder

Serve steaming bowls of this chowder with Whole-Grain Seed and Nut Bread (see recipe, page 186) and a salad for lunch or supper. Don't be afraid to experiment with the various mushrooms available in the supermarket. In fact, brown mushrooms such as cremini mushrooms give this soup a rich, mellow flavor.

MAKES ABOUT 6 CUPS (1.5 L)

MAKE AHEAD

Prepare through Step 1, ladle into an airtight container and store in the refrigerator for up to 2 days. Do not freeze.

2	slices bacon, diced	2
1	onion, chopped	1
1	stalk celery, diced	1
1	clove garlic, minced	1
8 oz	mushrooms, sliced	250 g
2 tsp	dried tarragon	10 mL
1 tbsp	all-purpose flour	15 mL
4 cups	Basic Chicken Stock (see recipe, page 68)	1 L
2	large potatoes, peeled and diced (about 2½ cups/625 mL)	2
½ cup	dry white wine	125 mL
½ tsp	salt	2 mL
½ tsp	freshly ground black pepper	2 mL
¼ cup	chopped fresh parsley	50 mL

1. In a large saucepan, over medium-low heat, cook bacon, onion, celery, garlic, mushrooms and tarragon, covered, for 5 to 8 minutes, or until onions are tender and mushrooms release liquid. Sprinkle with flour and stir in. Gradually whisk in chicken stock, stirring, until thickened and smooth. Add potatoes, wine, salt and pepper. Increase heat to medium, cover and cook until potatoes are tender, about 20 minutes.

2. Ladle into serving bowls and stir in parsley.

Nutritional value
Per serving (1 cup/250 mL)

Calories	147
Protein	7 g
Fat	3 g
Carbohydrate	21 g
Dietary Fiber (a source)	2 g
Calcium	44 mg

Percent of calories from

Protein	19%
Fat	17%
Carbohydrate	55%

Salmon Chowder

Sockeye salmon gives this chowder a lovely pink tinge, but any salmon will do. Remember to include the calcium-rich bones. Serve with Whole-Grain Seed and Nut Bread (see recipe, page 186).

MAKES ABOUT 8 CUPS (2 L)

MAKE AHEAD

Ladle into an airtight container and store in the refrigerator for up to 2 days. Do not freeze.

2 tbsp	vegetable oil	25 mL
1	onion, chopped	1
1	stalk celery, diced	1
1	carrot, peeled and diced	1
1	clove garlic, minced	1
2	potatoes, peeled and diced	2
4 cups	Basic Chicken Stock (see recipe, page 68)	1 L
1	can (7.5 oz/213 g) sockeye salmon	1
1 cup	dry white wine	250 mL
¼ cup	chopped fresh dill	50 mL
	Freshly ground black pepper	

1. In a large saucepan, heat oil over medium heat. Cook onion, celery, carrot and garlic, covered, for 8 to 10 minutes, or until softened but not browned. Stir in potatoes and chicken stock. Increase heat to high and bring to a boil; reduce heat to medium, cover and simmer until potatoes are tender, about 20 minutes.

2. Drain salmon; discard skin and mash bones. Add salmon and mashed bones, wine and dill to soup. Increase heat to high and bring to a boil. Season to taste with pepper.

Nutritional value
Per serving (1 cup/250 mL)

Calories	158
Protein	8 g
Fat	6 g
Carbohydrate	12 g
Dietary Fiber	1 g
Calcium (a source)	106 mg

Percent of calories from

Protein	21%
Fat	37%
Carbohydrate	30%

Creamy Clam Chowder

Even the lactose intolerant can enjoy this version of clam chowder. Add a crusty loaf and a salad, and you have a hearty meal for lunch or supper.

TIP

An easy way to cook bacon is in the microwave, wrapped in a paper towel on a microwave-safe plate. Cook 4 slices on High for 2 minutes. Cook vegetables in 2 tbsp (25 mL) vegetable oil instead of bacon fat.

4	slices side bacon, chopped	4
1	onion, chopped	1
1	leek, sliced	1
2	carrots, peeled and diced	2
2	potatoes, peeled and diced	2
1	clove garlic, minced	1
1	bay leaf	1
2 cups	Basic Chicken Stock (see recipe, page 68)	500 mL
1/2 tsp	hot pepper sauce	2 mL
1 to 2	cans (each 7 oz/184 mL) clams	1 to 2
2 cups	2% lactose-free milk or fortified soy milk	500 mL
	Chopped fresh parsley	

1. In a large saucepan or Dutch oven, over medium heat, cook bacon until crisp, about 5 minutes. Remove bacon to a plate, let cool and crumble.

2. In bacon fat, cook onion and leek, covered, until softened, about 5 minutes. Stir in carrots, potatoes, garlic, bay leaf, chicken stock and hot pepper sauce. Cook for 10 to 15 minutes, or until vegetables are tender. Stir in clams with their juice and milk. Simmer for 5 to 10 minutes, or until heated through.

3. Ladle into serving bowls and garnish with crumbled bacon and parsley.

Nutritional value
Per serving (1 cup/250 mL)

Calories	289
Protein	25 g
Fat	11 g
Carbohydrate	22 g
Dietary Fiber (a source)	2 g
Calcium (a source)	143 mg

Percent of calories from

Protein	35%
Fat	34%
Carbohydrate	31%

Salads

Salad dressings frequently use sour cream, buttermilk or sometimes cream cheese to give that luscious, rich texture and flavor. Again, silken soft tofu replaces these ingredients, and along with added herbs and seasonings it makes luxuriant sauces. You will find a food processor is a real asset to whipping up the dressings and creating the smooth texture.

These lactose-free salads incorporate tofu made with calcium chloride or calcium sulfate, vegetables containing calcium (see chart, page 22), additional herbs, beans (especially soybeans) and toasted nuts or seeds for taste, texture and added calcium. Don't forget to incorporate calcium greens — kale, broccoli, bok choy, collard greens, cabbage, napa cabbage and Chinese cabbage — into your salads.

Spring Salad with Oriental Flavors . . . 84

Greek Salad 85

Caesar Salad with Creamy
　　Garlic Dressing 86

Layered Salad with
　　Ranch-Style Dressing 88

Broccoli Apple Salad with
　　Creamy Curry Dressing 90

Salad of Fresh Spring Greens,
　　New Potatoes and Asparagus 92

Spinach, Almond and Orange Salad
　　with Creamy Tarragon Dressing . . . 94

Cucumber Almond Salad 96

French Potato Salad 97

Rossolye Salad 98

Salmon and Wild Rice Salad 100

Nice 'n' Nutty Slaw 102

Pasta Salad 104

Spring Salad with Oriental Flavors

Tofu and sesame seeds are sources of calcium. Any leftover tofu can be frozen for future use. For variety, feel free to substitute the best veggies available — sliced bok choy, broccoli, fiddleheads or mushrooms.

MAKES 6 SERVINGS

MAKE AHEAD

Dressing can be stored in an airtight container in the refrigerator for up to 2 days.

4	carrots, peeled and cut into julienne strips	4
1 lb	asparagus, tough ends removed	500 g
2 cups	frozen peas	500 mL
1	small red bell pepper, cut into strips	1
6 oz	extra-firm tofu, cubed	175 g
1 tbsp	toasted sesame seeds (see tip, page 90)	15 mL

Oriental Dressing

1	clove garlic, minced	1
3 tbsp	vegetable oil	50 mL
3 tbsp	freshly squeezed lemon juice	50 mL
2 tbsp	liquid honey	25 mL
2 tsp	grated gingerroot	10 mL
2 tsp	soy sauce	10 mL
1/4 tsp	salt	1 mL
Pinch	freshly ground black pepper	Pinch

1. In a large pot of boiling water, cook carrots, asparagus and peas for 2 to 3 minutes, or until tender-crisp. Drain and refresh under cold water.

2. *Prepare the Oriental Dressing:* In a small bowl, whisk together garlic, oil, lemon juice, honey, ginger, soy sauce, salt and pepper.

3. In a large bowl, toss asparagus, peas, carrots, red pepper and tofu with dressing just before serving. Sprinkle with sesame seeds.

Nutritional value	
Per serving	
Calories	188
Protein	8 g
Fat	9 g
Carbohydrate	21 g
Dietary Fiber (a high source)	4 g
Calcium (a source)	63 mg
Percent of calories from	
Protein	16%
Fat	42%
Carbohydrate	42%

Greek Salad

Naturally, Greek salad calls for feta cheese, made from goat's milk. Some lactose-intolerant people can digest feta more easily than cheese made from cow's milk. However, you will have to be the judge of whether this salad is right for you.

TIPS

Toss salad with dressing just before serving. For best flavor, serve at room temperature.

If fresh oregano is not available, use 1 tsp (5 mL) dried; crush between your fingers before adding to the dressing.

2	large ripe tomatoes, cut in 1-inch (2.5 cm) chunks	2
½	English cucumber, cut in thick slices	½
½	sweet onion, such as red or Vidalia, sliced	½
½ cup	Greek-style olives	125 mL
½ cup	feta cheese, crumbled (optional, if tolerated)	125 mL

Dressing

1	small clove garlic, crushed	1
⅓ cup	olive oil	75 mL
2 tbsp	red wine vinegar	25 ml
1 tbsp	chopped fresh oregano	15 mL
½ tsp	salt	2 mL
¼ tsp	freshly ground black pepper	1 mL

1. In a large bowl, combine tomatoes, cucumber, onion and olives.

2. *Prepare the dressing.* In a small bowl, whisk together garlic, oil, vinegar, oregano, garlic, salt and pepper until well combined.

3. Pour dressing over salad and toss gently. Crumble feta cheese (if using) over salad.

Variation

Add 2 cups (500 mL) chopped romaine lettuce or calcium greens such as sliced kale, napa cabbage or bok choy to the salad.

Dressing: Nutritional value Per Serving (1½ tbsp/22 mL)

Calories: 146, Protein: 0 g, Fat: 16 g, Carbohydrate: 1 g, Dietary Fiber: 0 g, Calcium: 7 mg

Percent of calories from
Protein: 8%, Fat: 98%, Carbohydrate: 1%

Salad with dressing
Nutritional value
Per serving

Calories	203
Protein	1 g
Fat	19 g
Carbohydrate	7 g
Dietary Fiber (a source)	2 g
Calcium	27 mg
Percent of calories from	
Protein	3%
Fat	84%
Carbohydrate	14%

Caesar Salad with Creamy Garlic Dressing

Probably the most popular salad on any menu, this version has plenty of zing with just a hint of cheese for flavor. If your tolerance to fresh Parmesan is low, substitute more croutons, a sprinkling of chopped sardines or chopped Salted Almonds (see recipe, page 49).

MAKES 4 SERVINGS

TIP

This recipe makes about twice as much creamy dressing as you need for the salad. Use the rest as a great dip for calcium-containing veggies, such as small kale leaves or broccoli florets.

1	head romaine lettuce	1
1 2/3 cups	Whole Wheat Croutons (see recipe, page 251)	400 mL
1 cup	freshly grated Parmesan cheese (optional, it tolerated)	250 mL
1/2 cup	chopped sardines or chopped sun-dried tomatoes	125 mL

Creamy Garlic Dressing

1	package (10.25 oz/290 g) silken soft tofu	1
1	clove garlic, minced	1
2 tbsp	freshly squeezed lemon juice	25 mL
1 tbsp	vegetable oil	15 mL
2 tsp	Dijon mustard	10 mL
1 tsp	salt	5 mL
1 tsp	granulated sugar	5 mL
1/4 tsp	freshly ground black pepper	1 mL
Pinch	cayenne pepper	Pinch

1. Tear lettuce into bite-size pieces. Cover and refrigerate until ready to toss. Sprinkle with croutons, cheese (if using) and sardines.

Salad with dressing
Nutritional value
Per serving

Calories	358
Protein	21 g
Fat	22 g
Carbohydrate	23 g
Dietary Fiber (a high source)	5 g
Calcium (a very high source)	475 mg

Percent of calories from

Protein	23%
Fat	53%
Carbohydrate	24%

2. *Prepare the Creamy Garlic Dressing:* Using a sieve, drain tofu. In a food processor, using pulsing action, purée tofu, garlic, lemon juice, oil, mustard, salt, sugar, pepper and cayenne.

3. Pour half of the dressing over salad (see tip, opposite) and toss to coat evenly.

Dressing: **Nutritional value** Per Serving (2 tbsp/25 mL)

Calories: 37, Protein: 2 g, Fat: 3 g, Carbohydrate: 2 g, Dietary Fiber: 0 g, Calcium: 13 mg

Percent of calories from
Protein: 18%, Fat: 61%, Carbohydrate: 21%

TIP

Instead of using all romaine lettuce, incorporate kale leaves or shredded napa cabbage into your Caesar salad for more calcium.

MAKE AHEAD

Salad can be prepared through Step 1, covered and stored in the refrigerator for up to 1 day. Dressing can be stored in an airtight container in the refrigerator for up to 2 days.

Layered Salad with Ranch-Style Dressing

This is truly a salad for all seasons because you can change the ingredients with the changing crops. It's a great salad for taking to potlucks or picnics, because it can be assembled ahead and tossed at the last minute. By including almonds and beans, you have a source of calcium, fiber and protein.

MAKES 8 SERVINGS

TIPS

For additional calcium, replace the spinach and romaine with shredded kale and napa cabbage.

Toasting nuts intensifies their flavor. To toast almonds, bake in preheated 350°F (180°C) oven for 10 to 12 minutes, or until golden brown and fragrant.

Salad with dressing	
Nutritional value	
Per serving	
Calories	130
Protein	8 g
Fat	6 g
Carbohydrate	15 g
Dietary Fiber (a high source)	5 g
Calcium (a source)	98 mg
Percent of calories from	
Protein	22%
Fat	37%
Carbohydrate	42%

1	package (10 oz/284 g) fresh spinach (or 1 head romaine), washed and dried	1
8 oz	mushrooms, sliced	250 g
1	red onion, thinly sliced	1
1	can (19 oz/284 mL) white or red kidney beans, drained	1
1	red bell pepper, chopped	1
2	stalks celery, sliced	2
½ cup	toasted coarsely chopped unblanched almonds (see tip, at left)	125 mL

Ranch-Style Dressing

1	package (10.25 oz/290 g) silken soft tofu	1
1	clove garlic, crushed	1
2 tbsp	light mayonnaise	25 mL
2 tbsp	white wine vinegar	25 mL
1 tbsp	granulated sugar	15 mL
1 tsp	salt	5 mL
¼ tsp	freshly ground black pepper	1 mL

1. Tear spinach into bite-size pieces; arrange half over the bottom of 9-inch (23 cm) salad bowl. Sprinkle evenly with half each of the mushrooms, red onion, beans, red pepper and celery. Repeat with another layer of spinach, mushrooms, red onion, beans, red pepper and celery.

2. *Prepare the Ranch-Style Dressing:* Using a sieve, drain tofu. In a food processor, using pulsing action, purée tofu, garlic, mayonnaise, vinegar, sugar, salt and pepper.

3. Spread dressing over top of salad. Sprinkle with almonds. To serve, spoon through layers so that each serving contains all ingredients.

Dressing: **Nutritional value** Per Serving (1 tbsp/15 mL)

Calories: 36, Protein: 2 g, Fat: 2 g, Carbohydrate: 3 g, Dietary Fiber: 0 g, Calcium: 13 mg

Percent of calories from
Protein: 19%, Fat: 45%, Carbohydrate: 36%

> ### MAKE AHEAD
> Cover and store in the refrigerator for up to 1 day.

Broccoli Apple Salad with Creamy Curry Dressing

A great winter salad with the calcium crunch of broccoli, this can also serve as a filling for pitas. Or add cooked chicken for a summer main course. The curried dressing makes a great dip for veggies too!

TIP

To toast sesame seeds, arrange on a baking sheet and bake in a 350°F (180°C) oven for 10 to 12 minutes, or until golden brown and fragrant.

1	bunch broccoli	1
3	apples, cored and coarsely chopped	3
2	stalks celery, sliced	2
1 cup	sunflower sprouts or alfalfa sprouts	250 mL
1/4 cup	toasted sesame seeds (see tip, at left)	50 mL

Creamy Curry Dressing

1	package (10.25 oz/290 g) silken soft tofu	1
2 tbsp	freshly squeezed lemon juice	25 mL
2 tbsp	vegetable oil	25 mL
1 tbsp	granulated sugar	15 mL
1 tsp	curry powder	5 mL
1 tsp	salt	5 mL
1/4 tsp	freshly ground black pepper	1 mL

1. Trim tough broccoli stems. Cut broccoli into florets and remaining stem into thin slices. In a pot of rapidly boiling water, cook broccoli, uncovered, for 4 to 5 minutes or until tender-crisp. Drain and run under cold water to stop broccoli cooking.

2. In a large bowl, combine broccoli, apples and celery.

Salad with dressing
Nutritional value
Per serving

Calories	131
Protein	5 g
Fat	7 g
Carbohydrate	16 g
Dietary Fiber (a high source)	4 g
Calcium (a source)	101 mg

Percent of calories from

Protein	13%
Fat	42%
Carbohydrate	45%

3. *Prepare the Creamy Curry Dressing:* Using a sieve, drain tofu. In a food processor, purée drained tofu, lemon juice, oil, sugar, curry powder, salt and pepper until smooth. Toss salad with enough dressing to lightly coat.

4. Serve on a bed of sunflower sprouts, garnished with sesame seeds.

Dressing: **Nutritional value** Per Serving (1 tbsp/15 mL)

Calories: 17, Protein: 1 g, Fat: 1 g, Carbohydrate: 1 g, Dietary Fiber: 0 g, Calcium: 5 mg

Percent of calories from
Protein: 13%, Fat: 65%, Carbohydrate: 22%

MAKE AHEAD

Dressing can be stored in an airtight container in the refrigerator for up to 2 days.

Salad of Fresh Spring Greens, New Potatoes and Asparagus

This beautiful salad is a true celebration of spring or summer.

MAKES 6 SERVINGS

TIPS

This salad is wonderful as a bed for grilled salmon. Sprinkle it with herbs and serve with lemon wedges.

For the best taste and freshness, choose asparagus with a bright green stalk and tightly closed, purple-tinged tips.

Salad with vinaigrette	
Nutritional value	
Per serving	
Calories	362
Protein	9 g
Fat	17 g
Carbohydrate	47 g
Dietary Fiber (a very high source)	6 g
Calcium (a high source)	176 mg
Percent of calories from	
Protein	10%
Fat	40%
Carbohydrate	50%

12	small new potatoes, scrubbed	12
1 lb	asparagus, tough ends removed	500 g
8 oz	fiddleheads	125 g
16 cups	assorted field greens (beet greens, watercress, Boston, leaf, romaine, arugula)	4 L
2	large hothouse tomatoes, cut in wedges	2

Herbal Vinaigrette

1	clove garlic, minced	1
1/4 cup	white wine vinegar	50 mL
1/4 cup	water	50 mL
1/4 cup	vegetable oil	50 mL
1/4 cup	extra-virgin olive oil	50 mL
2 tsp	chopped fresh tarragon, thyme or rosemary	10 mL
2 tsp	Dijon mustard	10 mL
1 tsp	salt	5 mL
1 tsp	granulated sugar	5 mL
1/4 tsp	freshly ground black pepper	1 mL

1. In a steamer over simmering water, steam potatoes until tender, about 15 minutes. Drain well.

2. Meanwhile, in a large pot of boiling water, cook asparagus and fiddleheads for 2 to 3 minutes, or until tender-crisp. Drain and refresh under cold water. Cut asparagus into 2-inch (10 cm) pieces.

3. *Prepare the Herbal Vinaigrette:* In a small bowl, whisk together garlic, vinegar, water, vegetable oil, olive oil, tarragon, mustard, salt, sugar and pepper until smooth.

4. In a large bowl, toss together greens, potatoes, asparagus and fiddleheads with enough dressing to coat. Arrange on a platter or individual plates. Garnish with tomato wedges.

Vinaigrette: **Nutritional value** Per Serving (1 tbsp/15 mL)

Calories: 58, Protein: 0 g, Fat: 6 g, Carbohydrate:1 g, Dietary Fiber: 0 g, Calcium: 10 mg

Percent of calories from
Protein: 1%, Fat: 94%, Carbohydrate: 6%

Tomato Basil Salad: Slice beefsteak or hothouse tomatoes and arrange on a platter. Drizzle with extra-virgin olive oil and sprinkle with chopped fresh basil and 2 cloves garlic, minced. Cover until ready to serve. Serve at room temperature.

TIPS

Choose fiddleheads that are tightly closed and bright green in color. Rinse them in several changes of water to remove any debris, then trim the root ends.

Instead of the field greens, try shredded calcium greens, such as kale, napa cabbage and Chinese cabbage.

Spinach, Almond and Orange Salad with Creamy Tarragon Dressing

This salad is the perfect accompaniment to chicken or fish dishes.

MAKES 6 SERVINGS

TIP

Toasting nuts intensifies their flavor. To toast almonds, bake in preheated 350°F (180°C) oven for 10 to 12 minutes, or until golden brown and fragrant.

1	package (10 oz/284 g) fresh spinach	1
2	seedless navel oranges	2
1/4	red onion, thinly sliced	1/4
1/2 cup	toasted chopped unblanched almonds (see tip, at left)	125 mL

Creamy Tarragon Dressing

1	package (10.25 oz/290 g) silken soft tofu	1
2 tbsp	light mayonnaise	25 mL
1 tbsp	white wine vinegar	15 mL
2 tsp	dried tarragon	10 mL
2 tsp	granulated sugar	10 mL
1 tsp	Dijon mustard	5 mL
1 tsp	salt	5 mL
1/4 tsp	freshly ground black pepper	1 mL

1. Trim spinach and tear into bite-size pieces. Using a sharp knife, cut away peel and white pith from oranges; slice crosswise into thin circles.

2. In a large salad bowl, combine spinach, orange slices and onion.

Salad with dressing
Nutritional value
Per serving

Calories	124
Protein	6 g
Fat	6 g
Carbohydrate	15 g
Dietary Fiber (a high source)	4 g
Calcium (a source)	124 mg

Percent of calories from

Protein	17%
Fat	39%
Carbohydrate	45%

3. *Prepare the Creamy Tarragon Dressing:* Using a sieve, drain tofu. In a blender or food processor, using pulsing motion, combine drained tofu, mayonnaise, vinegar, tarragon, sugar, mustard, salt and pepper until smooth. (Makes enough dressing for 2 salads.)

4. Toss salad with about half the dressing, or enough dressing to coat, and sprinkle with almonds.

Variation

For added calcium, substitute shredded calcium greens such as napa cabbage or kale for the spinach.

Dressing: **Nutritional value** Per Serving (1 tbsp/15 mL)

Calories: 47, Protein: 3 g, Fat: 3 g, Carbohydrate: 4 g, Dietary Fiber: 0 g, Calcium: 23 mg

Percent of calories from
Protein: 21%, Fat: 47%, Carbohydrate: 32%

MAKE AHEAD

Salad can be assembled through Step 2, covered and stored in the refrigerator for up to 4 hours. Dressing can be stored in an airtight container in the refrigerator for up to 2 days. Toss salad with dressing just before serving.

Cucumber Almond Salad

The calcium crunch from the almonds is a delectable contrast to the freshness of the cucumber. The salad is a great partner to fish or seafood. Try the luscious dressing over shredded calcium greens, such as napa cabbage, Chinese cabbage or bok choy.

MAKES 6 SERVINGS

TIPS

Almonds go soggy if combined in a salad with dressing and allowed to stand.

Toasting nuts intensifies their flavor. To toast almonds, bake in preheated 350°F (180°C) oven for 10 to 12 minutes, or until golden brown and fragrant.

Dressing

1 tsp	grated lemon zest	5 mL
¼ cup	freshly squeezed lemon juice	50 mL
¼ cup	vegetable oil	50 mL
1 tbsp	liquid honey	15 mL
½ tsp	salt	2 mL
¼ tsp	freshly ground black pepper	1 mL
1	English cucumber, thinly sliced (about ⅛ inch/3 mm)	1
½ cup	toasted slivered unblanched almonds (see tip, at left)	125 mL

1. *Prepare the dressing:* In a small bowl or food processor, combine lemon zest, lemon juice, oil, honey, salt and pepper.

2. Place cucumbers in a large bowl and toss with enough dressing to coat. (You may have enough for 2 salads, depending on size of cucumber.) Sprinkle with almonds.

Nutritional value
Per serving

Calories	152
Protein	3 g
Fat	13 g
Carbohydrate	9 g
Dietary Fiber (a source)	2 g
Calcium	44 mg

Percent of calories from

Protein	6%
Fat	72%
Carbohydrate	22%

French Potato Salad

An early summer treat, this tastes wonderful with tiny garden-fresh new potatoes. Instead of the usual creamy mayo-dressed potato salad, try this tangy marinade that's free of dairy — making it safe to tote on picnics.

MAKES 8 SERVINGS

MAKE AHEAD

Cover and store in the refrigerator for up to 2 days.

2 lbs	tiny new potatoes or quartered larger potatoes (8 cups/2 L)	1 kg

Marinade

½ cup	vegetable oil	125 ml
¼ cup	white wine vinegar	50 mL
¼ cup	white wine	50 mL
1 tsp	Dijon mustard	5 mL
1 tsp	salt	5 mL
1 tsp	dried tarragon	5 mL
¼ tsp	freshly ground black pepper	1 mL
2 tbsp	chopped fresh parsley	25 mL
2 tbsp	chopped fresh chives	25 mL

1. Scrub but do not peel potatoes. Steam for 15 to 20 minutes, until tender. Transfer to a large bowl.

2. *Prepare the marinade:* In a small bowl, whisk together oil, vinegar, wine, mustard, salt, tarragon and pepper. Pour over warm potatoes.

3. Sprinkle potatoes with parsley and chives, toss gently. Serve at room temperature.

Nutritional value
Per serving

Calories	243
Protein	3 g
Fat	15 g
Carbohydrate	26 g
Dietary Fiber (a source)	2 g
Calcium	13 mg

Percent of calories from

Protein	4%
Fat	53%
Carbohydrate	42%

Rossolye Salad

This colorful Russian beet and apple salad with sardines is a tasty addition to a buffet table. The sardines and the dressing both contain calcium. The dressing can do triple duty as a sauce for fish, a spread for sandwiches or a vegetable dip.

MAKES 6 SERVINGS

TIPS

In the spring, beets are sold with their leaves attached. Choose regular, blemish-free beets and store them in a plastic bag in the vegetable crisper for 2 to 3 days. Winter beets are sold without their leaves and may be stored in a plastic bag in the vegetable crisper for up to 1 week.

One lemon will yield about 3 tbsp (25 mL) of juice.

Salad with dressing
Nutritional value
Per serving

Calories	176
Protein	8 g
Fat	5 g
Carbohydrate	27 g
Dietary Fiber (a source)	3 g
Calcium (a source)	109 mg
Percent of calories from	
Protein	17%
Fat	25%
Carbohydrate	59%

1	bunch beets, washed	1
3	potatoes, peeled and quartered	3
2	apples, cored and coarsely chopped	2
1	can (3.75 oz/100 g) sardines, drained and chopped	1
	Dill sprigs	

Creamy Dill Dressing

1	package (10.25 oz/290 g) silken soft tofu	1
1/3 cup	chopped fresh dill	75 mL
3 tbsp	freshly squeezed lemon juice	45 mL
2 tbsp	vegetable oil	25 mL
1 tbsp	Dijon mustard	15 mL
1 tbsp	granulated sugar	15 mL
1 tsp	salt	5 mL
1/4 tsp	freshly ground black pepper	1 mL

1. In a large pot of rapidly boiling water, cook beets, uncovered, until tender, about 20 minutes. Drain and let cool enough to handle. Peel and dice into 1/2-inch (1 cm) cubes.

2. In same pot with more water, cook potatoes until tender, about 15 minutes. Drain and dice into 1/2-inch (1 cm) cubes.

3. In a large bowl, combine cooled beets, potatoes and apples. Set aside.

4. *Prepare the Creamy Dill Dressing:* Using a sieve, drain tofu. In a food processor, using pulsing action, purée drained tofu, dill, lemon juice, oil, mustard, sugar, salt and pepper.

5. Toss salad gently with about half of the dressing, or just enough to coat. Serve garnished with sardines and dill. Pass bowl of remaining dressing separately.

Dressing: Nutritional value Per Serving (2 tbsp/25 mL)

Calories: 58, Protein: 2 g, Fat: 4 g, Carbohydrate: 3 g, Dietary Fiber: 0 g, Calcium: 13 mg

Percent of calories from
Protein: 12%, Fat: 67%, Carbohydrate: 21%

MAKE AHEAD

Salad can be covered and stored in the refrigerator for up to 1 day. Dressing can be stored in an airtight container in the refrigerator for up to 2 days.

Salmon and Wild Rice Salad

Try this salad throughout the seasons, varying the vegetables with the freshest ones available. Canned salmon with the bones is an excellent source of calcium and vitamin D, essential for the absorption of calcium. Be sure to mash the bones and add them to the salad for added calcium. When you accompany this with good bread, such as Whole-Grain Seed and Nut Bread (see recipe, page 186) or Double Cornbread (see recipe, page 188), and a green salad in spring or summer or a hearty soup in fall or winter, you have a satisfying meal.

MAKES 6 SERVINGS

TIP

Peas, asparagus spears, green beans, fiddleheads or sliced zucchini may be substituted for the broccoli florets. To prepare asparagus, break off tough root end. Slice zucchini; leave green beans whole but cut off ends. Fiddleheads are the tightly coiled emerging fronds of the ostrich fern. They need

Nutritional value
Per serving

Calories	550
Protein	22 g
Fat	28 g
Carbohydrate	56 g
Dietary Fiber (a source)	3 g
Calcium (a high source)	232 mg

Percent of calories from

Protein	16%
Fat	45%
Carbohydrate	40%

1 cup	wild rice	250 mL
5 cups	water, divided	1.25 L
1 ½ tsp	salt, divided	7 mL
2	bay leaves	2
1 cup	long-grain parboiled rice	250 mL
1 lb	broccoli florets	500 g
2	cans (each 7.5 oz/213 g) sockeye salmon	2
8 oz	whole button mushrooms	250 g
½ cup	chopped fresh parsley	125 mL
4	green onions, chopped	4
½	red bell pepper, chopped	½

Dressing

1	clove garlic, minced	1
½ cup	vegetable oil	125 mL
¼ cup	red wine vinegar	50 mL
1 tbsp	granulated sugar	15 mL
½ tsp	salt	2 mL
¼ tsp	freshly ground black pepper	1 mL

1. Rinse wild rice and cover with cold water. Let soak for 30 minutes. Drain.

2. In a large saucepan, bring 3 cups (750 mL) of the water, 1 tsp (5 mL) of the salt and 1 of the bay leaves to a boil over high heat. Stir in wild rice; bring back to boil. Reduce heat to medium and cook, covered, until tender, about 25 minutes. Drain and let cool. Discard bay leaf.

3. In a medium saucepan, bring the remaining water, the remaining salt and the remaining bay leaf to a boil over high heat. Add parboiled rice; reduce heat to medium and simmer, covered, for 15 minutes. Remove from heat and let stand, covered, for 5 minutes, or until all liquid is absorbed. Let cool. Discard bay leaf.

4. Meanwhile, in a large pot of rapidly boiling salted water, cook broccoli, uncovered, until tender-crisp, about 2 to 3 minutes. Drain and refresh under cold water.

5. Drain salmon; discard skin and mash bones. In a large bowl, combine cooled wild and parboiled rice, broccoli, salmon with mashed bones, mushrooms, parsley, green onions and red pepper.

6. *Prepare the dressing:* In a small bowl, whisk together garlic, oil, vinegar, sugar, salt and pepper. Pour over salad and toss gently.

to be rinsed in several changes of water to remove any debris. Trim root end. All green vegetables should be cooked uncovered to maintain their bright green color.

MAKE AHEAD

Cover and store in the refrigerator for up to 1 day.

Nice 'n' Nutty Slaw

Used instead of the usual creamy coleslaw dressing, this oil-and-vinegar version allows you to marinate the slaw for several hours. It is a colorful addition to potlucks or picnics. Calcium is boosted with the crunch of sesame seeds, sprouts and almonds. Feel free to experiment with your own combination of shredded vegetables; try including some of those containing calcium (see page 22).

MAKES 8 SERVINGS

TIPS

Fennel is a slightly sweet licorice-flavored vegetable with the crunch of celery. If you have difficulty finding it in your local supermarket, look in an Italian fruit and vegetable store.

Experiment with other calcium-containing cabbages, such as napa and Chinese cabbage.

Nutritional value
Per serving

Calories	118
Protein	5 g
Fat	7 g
Carbohydrate	13 g
Dietary Fiber (a high source)	5 g
Calcium (a source)	146 mg
Percent of calories from	
Protein	14%
Fat	46%
Carbohydrate	40%

● Preheat oven to 350°F (180°C)
● Baking sheet

1/2 cup	sliced unblanched almonds	125 mL
1/4 cup	sesame seeds	50 mL
3	green onions, sliced	3
3 cups	shredded red cabbage	750 mL
3 cups	shredded green cabbage	750 mL
2 cups	sunflower sprouts or alfalfa sprouts	500 mL
1 cup	sliced fennel or celery	250 mL
1/2 cup	chopped fresh parsley	125 mL
1	apple, cored and sliced	1

Poppy Seed Dressing

1/4 cup	white wine vinegar or freshly squeezed lemon juice	50 mL
2 tbsp	chopped onion	25 mL
2 tbsp	granulated sugar	25 mL
1 tbsp	poppy seeds	15 mL
1/2 tsp	salt	2 mL
1/4 tsp	freshly ground black pepper	1 mL
1/4 cup	vegetable oil	50 mL

1. Spread almonds and sesame seeds on baking sheet. Bake in preheated oven for 10 to 12 minutes, or until golden brown. Let cool.

2. In a large bowl, combine onions, red and green cabbage, sprouts, fennel, and parsley.

3. *Prepare the Poppy Seed Dressing:* In a small bowl, whisk together vinegar, onion, sugar, poppy seeds, salt and pepper. Whisk in oil.

4. Up to 4 hours before serving, toss almonds, sesame seeds and apples with cabbage mixture; toss with dressing until well mixed. (Longer marinating will cause apples to brown and almonds to become soggy.)

Variation

Substitute an equal amount of bok choy for the fennel. It adds a wonderful calcium crunch!

MAKE AHEAD

Salad can be prepared through Step 2, covered and stored in the refrigerator for up to 1 day. Dressing can be stored in an airtight container in the refrigerator for up to 2 weeks.

Pasta Salad

Many pasta salads have cheese added for flavor. This version relies on a zesty dressing, instead. Soybeans add calcium and protein to this main-course salad.

TIP

Pasta absorbs flavor, so be sure to use a zesty dressing.

MAKE AHEAD

Prepare through Step 3, cover and store in the refrigerator for up to 1 day. Or prepare entire recipe, cover and store in the refrigerator for up to 4 hours.

8 oz	rotini or penne pasta	250 g
8 oz	green beans or broccoli	250 g
4	green onions, chopped	4
2	stalks celery, sliced	2
1	red bell pepper, thinly sliced	1
1	can (19 oz/540 mL) soybeans, drained and rinsed	1
2 cups	black or green olives, sliced	500 mL

Dressing

1	clove garlic, minced	1
1 cup	olive oil	250 mL
½ cup	chopped fresh parsley	125 mL
½ cup	white wine vinegar	125 mL
1 tbsp	granulated sugar	15 mL
1 tbsp	dried basil	15 mL
1 tsp	salt	5 mL
½ tsp	freshly ground black pepper	2 mL

1. In a large pot of boiling water, cook pasta until al dente (tender but firm to the bite), about 12 minutes. Immediately drain and rinse under cold water. Set aside.

2. In a large pot of boiling water, cook green beans until tender-crisp, about 7 minutes. Drain.

3. In a large bowl, combine pasta, green beans, onions, celery, red pepper, soybeans and olives. Set aside.

4. *Prepare the dressing:* In a medium bowl, whisk together garlic, oil, parsley, vinegar, sugar, basil, salt and pepper until well combined.

5. Pour dressing over salad and toss to coat.

Dressing: Nutritional value Per Serving (2 tbsp/25 mL)

Calories: 165, Protein: 0 g, Fat: 18 g, Carbohydrate: 1 g, Dietary Fiber: 0 g, Calcium: 10 mg
Percent of calories from
Protein: 0%, Fat: 96%, Carbohydrate: 3%

Salad with dressing
Nutritional value
Per serving

Calories	521
Protein	13 g
Fat	35 g
Carbohydrate	41 g
Dietary Fiber (a very high source)	6 g
Calcium (a source)	131 mg

Percent of calories from

Protein	10%
Fat	59%
Carbohydrate	31%

Pasta and Pizza

Pasta and pizza frequently include cheese toppings or cream sauces with accompanying bowls of cheese. By using a minimum of Parmesan cheese — an aged hard cheese — seasoned bread crumbs for topping and rich sauces made from lactose-free milk, pasta and pizza can still appear on the menu. Those with lactose intolerance will have to find their individual tolerance level for cheese. Aged hard cheeses, such as Parmesan, Gouda, Cheddar and Swiss, which are low in lactose, may be digested comfortably, especially if consumed in small quantities.

Pasta with Calcium Greens
and Almonds 106

Creamy Leek and Tomato Pasta 108

Pesto Pasta 109

Far East Noodles 110

Linguine with Creamy Mushroom
and Ham Sauce 112

Fettuccini Alfredo 113

Macaroni and Cheese 114

Tuna Noodle Casserole 116

Lazy Lasagna 118

Garden Lasagna 120

Florentine Lasagna 122

Margherita Pizza 124

Pesto Pizza 125

Bruschetta Pizza 126

Roasted Ratatouille Pizza 128

Four Onion Pizza with Rosemary . . . 130

Pasta with Calcium Greens and Almonds

Broccoli, kale and almonds give a calcium zing to this vibrant pasta dish.

TIPS

Clean mushrooms with a damp cloth. Do not immerse them in water — they soak up water like a sponge.

Store fresh mushrooms in the refrigerator for up to 1 week in a paper bag rather than in plastic, where they are too moist and become slimy.

If fresh tarragon and thyme are not available, substitute 1 tsp (5 mL) dried.

Nutritional value	
Per serving	
Calories	406
Protein	15 g
Fat	11 g
Carbohydrate	64 g
Dietary Fiber (a high source)	5 g
Calcium (a high source)	185 mg
Percent of calories from	
Protein	14%
Fat	24%
Carbohydrate	62%

4 cups	coarsely chopped kale, stems removed	1 L
2 cups	broccoli florets	500 mL
4 cups	fusilli pasta	1 L
2 tbsp	olive oil	25 mL
2	cloves garlic, minced	2
4 oz	sliced mushrooms	125 g
1	red bell pepper, cut in strips	1
2 tbsp	minced fresh tarragon	25 mL
2 tbsp	minced fresh thyme	25 mL
2 tbsp	balsamic vinegar	25 mL
½ tsp	salt	2 mL
¼ tsp	freshly ground black pepper	1 mL
½ cup	toasted unblanched almonds (see tips, opposite)	125 mL
½ cup	chopped green onions	125 mL

1. In a large pot of boiling water, cook kale until wilted, about 5 minutes. Drain, rinse under cold water and press out excess moisture. Set aside.

2. In a medium pot of boiling water, cook broccoli for 3 minutes, or until tender-crisp. Rinse under cold water; drain. Add to kale.

3. In a large pot of boiling salted water, cook fusilli for 8 to 10 minutes, or until al dente (tender but firm to the bite). Drain and set aside.

4. Meanwhile, in a large saucepan, heat oil over medium-high heat. Cook garlic and mushrooms, stirring, for 2 minutes. Add red pepper; cook, stirring, for 2 minutes. Add kale and broccoli; cook for 1 minute, or until heated through. Remove from heat and stir in tarragon, thyme, vinegar, salt and pepper.

5. Toss pasta with vegetables. Serve hot or at room temperature, garnished with almonds and green onions.

Variation

Substitute rotini or penne pasta for fusilli.

TIPS

Unblanched almonds have their skins on and appear brown. Blanched almonds, without skins, are white. Unblanched almonds maintain freshness better than blanched almonds.

Toasting nuts intensifies their flavor. To toast almonds, bake in preheated 350°F (180°C) oven for 10 to 12 minutes, or until golden brown and fragrant.

Creamy Leek and Tomato Pasta

Leeks are abundant during the winter months and jazz up weekday meals. Remember, they need careful washing because they are grown in sand, making their inner layers gritty.

MAKES 4 SERVINGS

TIPS

The easiest way to clean leeks is to chop off the tough green stem, leaving the white tender root. Slit this lengthwise almost to the root end, then wash under cold running water.

Cook pasta according to package directions. Allow 12 oz to 1 lb (375 to 500 g) pasta for 4 servings.

2 tbsp	extra-virgin olive oil	25 mL
3	leeks (white parts only), sliced thinly	3
2	tomatoes	2
1 tsp	dried oregano	5 mL
1/4 tsp	dried sage	1 mL
2 tbsp	all-purpose flour	25 mL
1 cup	chicken stock	250 mL
1 cup	lactose-free milk	250 mL
	Salt and freshly ground black pepper	
	Cooked rigatoni, fusilli or radiatore pasta	
	Freshly grated Parmesan cheese (optional, if tolerated)	

1. In a large saucepan, heat oil over medium heat. Cook leeks, covered, for 3 to 5 minutes, or until softened.

2. Meanwhile, in a large bowl, cover tomatoes with boiling water. Let stand for about 3 minutes. Drain and run under cold water; slip off skins. Cut each tomato into 8 wedges.

3. Sprinkle oregano and sage over leeks; stir in. Sprinkle with flour; cook, stirring, until flour is pale brown. Gradually whisk in chicken stock; cook, stirring until thickened. Stir in milk, tomatoes, and salt and pepper to taste; cook until heated through.

4. Toss pasta with sauce and serve sprinkled with cheese (if using).

Nutritional value
Per serving

Calories	742
Protein	25 g
Fat	11 g
Carbohydrate	134 g
Dietary Fiber (a very high source)	9 g
Calcium (a source)	144 mg

Percent of calories from

Protein	14%
Fat	14%
Carbohydrate	73%

Pesto Pasta

For an instant gourmet dinner, serve this emergency pasta dish with a green salad, hot crusty bread and chilled crisp white wine. You can't go wrong!

MAKES 4 SERVINGS

12 oz	fusilli pasta	375 g
	Parsley Pesto (see recipe, page 27)	
1 cup	freshly grated Parmesan cheese (optional, if tolerated)	250 mL

1. In a large saucepan of boiling salted water, cook pasta for 8 to 10 minutes, or until al dente (tender but firm to the bite).
2. Drain and toss with pesto. Serve with cheese (if using).

Nutritional value
Per serving

Calories	565
Protein	24 g
Fat	22 g
Carbohydrate	67 g
Dietary Fiber (a high source)	5 g
Calcium (a very high source)	445 mg

Percent of calories from

Protein	17%
Fat	36%
Carbohydrate	48%

Far East Noodles

Speedy enough for a weeknight meal, this exotic "dinner in a dish" can double as buffet fare. Extra-firm tofu, sesame seeds, broccoli and bok choy all contribute to the calcium content in this recipe. If your taste buds like more kick, spice up the dish with a dash or two of Chinese chili sauce.

MAKES 4 SERVINGS

TIPS

A rasp (available at cookware stores) works well to grate gingerroot.

Look for pre-cooked Cantonese noodles in the refrigerator counter of the meat or deli section of the grocery store.

To toast sesame seeds, arrange on a baking sheet and bake in a 350°F (180°C) oven for 10 to 12 minutes, or until golden brown and fragrant.

Nutritional value
Per serving

Calories	625
Protein	28 g
Fat	15 g
Carbohydrate	95 g
Dietary Fiber (a very high source)	6 g
Calcium (a high source)	261 mg

Percent of calories from

Protein	18%
Fat	21%
Carbohydrate	59%

8 oz	asparagus	250 g
2 cups	broccoli florets	500 mL
2 tbsp	vegetable oil	25 mL
12 oz	chicken breast or pork tenderloin, cut into strips	375 g
12 oz	extra-firm tofu, cut into 1/2-inch (1 cm) cubes	375 g
6	green onions, chopped	6
2	cloves garlic, crushed	2
1/2	red bell pepper, sliced	1/2
8 oz	mushrooms, sliced	250 g
2 cups	sliced bok choy	500 mL
2 tbsp	grated gingerroot	25 mL
1	package (12 oz/375 g) pre-cooked Cantonese noodles	1
2 tbsp	toasted sesame seeds (see tip, at left)	25 mL
2 tbsp	chopped fresh cilantro	25 mL

Sauce

1/2 cup	chicken stock (store-bought or see recipe, page 68)	125 mL
1/4 cup	dry sherry or rice wine vinegar	50 mL
3 tbsp	soy sauce	45 mL
2 tsp	cornstarch	10 mL
1 tsp	sesame oil	5 mL

1. Wash asparagus and break off tough ends; cut stalks into 2-inch (5 cm) diagonal pieces.

2. In a Dutch oven or wok, heat about 1 inch (2.5 cm) water to boiling. Add asparagus and broccoli; cook, uncovered, until tender-crisp, about 2 minutes. Drain and set aside.

3. In the same pan, heat oil over medium-high heat. Cook chicken until lightly brown and no longer pink inside, about 2 minutes. Sprinkle with asparagus mixture, tofu cubes, onions, garlic, red pepper, mushrooms, bok choy and ginger; cover and keep warm while preparing sauce.

4. *Prepare the sauce:* In a measuring cup, whisk together chicken stock, sherry, soy sauce, cornstarch and sesame oil.

5. Pour sauce over mixture in pan. Bring to a boil over medium-high heat; reduce heat to low and simmer, uncovered, for 2 to 3 minutes, or until sauce has thickened slightly and vegetables are tender-crisp. Stir mixture to coat with sauce.

6. Meanwhile, bring a kettleful of water to a boil. Pull noodles apart and place in a large bowl. Pour boiling water over noodles and let stand for 4 to 5 minutes, or until tender. Drain

7. Arrange noodles on a platter or individual serving dishes. Spoon meat mixture over noodles. Sprinkle with sesame seeds and cilantro.

TIP

Cilantro is also called Chinese parsley or coriander. It has a distinctive fragrance and taste that some people love and some people hate. If you are one of those who dislikes this herb, substitute chopped fresh parsley.

Linguine with Creamy Mushroom and Ham Sauce

This is a favorite in our house because it's quick and simple to make and has a wonderful richness, like cream, but with very little fat. It's special enough to serve for company.

MAKES 4 SERVINGS

TIP

Cook pasta according to package directions. Allow 12 oz to 1 lb (375 to 500 g) pasta for 4 servings.

2 tbsp	extra-virgin olive oil	25 mL
1	onion, chopped	1
1	clove garlic, minced	1
12 oz	mushrooms, sliced	375 g
1/4 cup	dry sherry or white wine	50 mL
1 tsp	dried thyme	5 mL
1/4 tsp	ground nutmeg	1 mL
2 tbsp	all-purpose flour	25 mL
2 cups	lactose-free milk or fortified soy milk	500 mL
1 cup	chopped Black Forest ham or smoked turkey	250 mL
1/4 cup	chopped fresh parsley	50 mL
1/2 tsp	salt	2 mL
1/4 tsp	freshly ground black pepper	1 mL
	Cooked linguine pasta	

1. In a large skillet, heat oil over medium heat; cook onion and garlic for 5 to 8 minutes, or until softened. Add mushrooms, sherry, thyme and nutmeg; cook, uncovered, until mushrooms release juices, about 5 minutes. Sprinkle with flour, stirring to combine. Gradually whisk in milk; cook, stirring, until smooth and thickened. Stir in ham, parsley, salt and pepper.

2. Toss pasta with sauce and serve immediately.

Nutritional value
Per serving

Calories	671
Protein	29 g
Fat	15 g
Carbohydrate	102 g
Dietary Fiber (a very high source)	6 g
Calcium (a high source)	204 mg

Percent of calories from

Protein	17%
Fat	19%
Carbohydrate	61%

Fettuccini Alfredo

To me, this is the ultimate luxury food — fast, rich and soothing. This lactose-free version is lower in fat than the original made with whipping cream, a bonus to be enjoyed without guilt!

MAKES 4 SERVINGS

2 tbsp	extra-virgin olive oil	25 mL
1	shallot, chopped	1
1	clove garlic, minced	1
2 tbsp	all-purpose flour	25 mL
2½ cups	2% lactose-free milk	625 mL
1	bay leaf	1
½ tsp	salt	2 mL
¼ tsp	freshly ground black pepper	1 mL
¼ tsp	ground nutmeg	1 mL
12 oz	fettuccini	375 g
	Freshly grated Parmesan cheese (optional, if tolerated)	

1. In a large saucepan, heat oil over medium heat; cook shallot and garlic until softened, about 5 minutes. Sprinkle with flour; cook, stirring, until pale brown, about 3 minutes. Remove from heat.

2. Meanwhile, in a separate saucepan, heat milk and bay leaf over medium heat until bubbles appear around edge of pan, about 4 minutes. Gradually whisk about half into shallot mixture until smooth and thickened.

3. Return shallot mixture to medium heat. Gradually whisk in remaining milk; cook, stirring, until thickened. Whisk in salt, pepper and nutmeg. Discard bay leaf.

4. In a large pot of boiling salted water, cook fettuccini for 6 to 8 minutes, or until al dente (tender but firm to the bite). Drain and toss with sauce. Serve sprinkled with cheese (if using).

Nutritional value
Per serving

Calories	460
Protein	17 g
Fat	11 g
Carbohydrate	75 g
Dietary Fiber (a source)	2 g
Calcium (a high source)	208 mg

Percent of calories from

Protein	14%
Fat	22%
Carbohydrate	64%

Macaroni and Cheese

Warm and comforting, macaroni and cheese is as popular with toddlers as with adults. Lactose-free milk adds natural sweetness and creaminess to the dish. Aged firm cheeses, such as Cheddar, Swiss, Gouda and Parmesan, are often better digested by lactose-intolerant people because they are low in lactose. Use only if tolerated.

MAKES 4 SERVINGS, ABOUT 6 CUPS (1.5 L)

TIPS

Using hot milk to make the béchamel sauce speeds up its thickening and makes it easier to keep smooth.

Fortified soy milk can be used instead of lactose-free milk to make the béchamel sauce. However, the flavor is flat, and the beige color requires more parsley.

Nutritional value
Per serving

Calories	769
Protein	36 g
Fat	37 g
Carbohydrate	70 g
Dietary Fiber (a source)	2 g
Calcium (a very high source)	344 mg

Percent of calories from

Protein	19%
Fat	44%
Carbohydrate	37%

- Preheat oven to 350°F (180°C)
- 6-cup (1.5 L) baking dish, greased

2 cups	elbow macaroni	500 mL
1 tsp	salt	5 mL

Béchamel Sauce

4 cups	lactose-free milk	1 L
1	bay leaf	1
1/4 cup	vegetable oil	50 mL
1/4 cup	all-purpose flour	50 mL
2 tsp	Dijon mustard	10 mL
2 tsp	Worcestershire sauce	10 mL
	Salt and freshly ground black pepper	
2 cups	shredded old Cheddar cheese (optional, if tolerated)	500 mL

Bread Crumb Topping

1/4 cup	dry bread crumbs	50 mL
1 tbsp	extra-virgin olive oil	15 mL
1 tbsp	freshly grated Parmesan cheese (optional, if tolerated)	15 mL
1 tbsp	chopped fresh parsley	15 mL

1. In a large pot of boiling water, cook macaroni and salt for 8 minutes, or until al dente (tender but firm to the bite). Drain.

2. *Meanwhile, prepare the Béchamel Sauce:* In a medium saucepan, heat milk and bay leaf over medium heat until bubbles appear around edge of pan, about 4 minutes.

3. Meanwhile, in a large saucepan, heat oil over medium heat. Stir in flour and cook until it starts to turn pale brown and pull away from side of pan. Gradually whisk in heated milk; cook until thickened and smooth, about 5 minutes. Whisk in mustard and Worcestershire sauce. Season with salt and pepper to taste. Stir in cheese (if using). Discard bay leaf.

4. Stir in macaroni until combined. Spoon into prepared baking dish.

5. *Prepare the Bread Crumb Topping:* In a small bowl, stir together bread crumbs, oil, cheese (if using) and parsley; sprinkle evenly over macaroni.

6. Bake in preheated oven for 30 to 35 minutes, or until bubbly and browned on top.

TIP

If Cheddar cheese is not tolerated in the quantity suggested in the recipe, substitute 1/4 cup to 1/2 cup (50 mL to 125 mL) freshly grated Parmesan cheese, depending on your tolerance level.

No-Fuss Mac and Cheese

In a large pot of boiling water, cook 1 1/2 cups (375 mL) elbow macaroni for 5 to 7 minutes, or until al dente (tender but firm to the bite). Drain. In the same pot, combine 1 cup (250 mL) lactose-free milk or fortified soy milk and 1 tbsp (15 mL) cornstarch. Cook over medium heat until thickened, about 2 minutes. Stir in macaroni and 3/4 cup (175 mL) shredded old Cheddar cheese or lactose-free Cheddar cheese until cheese is melted. Serve immediately. Makes 2 servings. (For a different twist, stir in 1/4 cup (50 mL) salsa and 2 cups (500 mL) blanched broccoli florets or calcium greens, such as kale, shredded napa cabbage or bok choy.)

Nutritional value Per Serving

Calories: 508, Protein: 24 g, Fat: 17 g, Carbohydrate: 65 g, Dietary Fiber: 2 g (a source), Calcium: 471 mg (a very high source)

Percent of calories from
Protein: 19%, Fat: 30%, Carbohydrate: 51%

Tuna Noodle Casserole

Considered comfort food by some, this popular casserole is designed with the lactose intolerant in mind.

TIPS

By using homemade chicken stock, you will be including some calcium in this dish. However, for convenience, you may wish to use a good commercial variety.

Use a blender or food processor to make fresh bread crumbs from sliced bread. For this recipe, you'll need about 2 slices.

Nutritional value
Per serving

Calories	461
Protein	24 g
Fat	19 g
Carbohydrate	51 g
Dietary Fiber (a very high source)	6 g
Calcium (a source)	145 mg

Percent of calories from

Protein	21%
Fat	36%
Carbohydrate	44%

- Preheat oven to 350°F (180°C)
- 8-cup (2 L) ovenproof casserole dish, sprayed with nonstick cooking spray

6 oz	egg noodles	175 g
1	can (6.5 oz/184 g) tuna packed in water, drained	1
4	green onions, sliced	4
1	stalk celery, chopped	1
½	red bell pepper, chopped	½
1 cup	Basic Chicken Stock (see recipe, page 68)	250 mL
¼ cup	light whipped salad dressing	50 mL
½ tsp	freshly ground black pepper	2 mL
½ tsp	dried tarragon	2 mL

Topping

1 cup	fresh bread crumbs (see tip, at left)	250 mL
½ cup	chopped unblanched almonds	125 mL
1 tbsp	vegetable oil	15 mL

1. In a large pot of boiling salted water, cook noodles until al dente (tender but firm to the bite), about 8 minutes. Drain and rinse under cold water.

2. In a large bowl, combine cooled noodles, tuna, green onions, celery and red pepper.

3. In a measuring cup, whisk together chicken stock, salad dressing, pepper and tarragon until well combined. Pour over noodle mixture and combine. Spoon into prepared casserole dish.

4. *Prepare the topping:* In a small bowl, toss bread crumbs, almonds and vegetable oil. Sprinkle evenly over top of casserole.

5. Bake in preheated oven for 30 to 35 minutes, or until heated through.

Variation

For a calcium-rich dish, substitute canned salmon with mashed bones for the tuna and add ½ cup to 1 cup (125 to 250 mL) calcium greens, such as blanched broccoli, kale or bok choy.

TIP

Unblanched almonds have their skins on and appear brown. Blanched almonds, without skins, are white. Unblanched almonds maintain freshness better than blanched almonds.

Lazy Lasagna

Who doesn't like lasagna? It's usually off-limits to the lactose intolerant, but not with this simple recipe!

TIPS

Béchamel sauce is often called a "mother" sauce. This means that it is a foundation for numerous other sauces, used in countless casseroles and dishes. Béchamel sauce is also called cream sauce.

To save time, heat the milk for the béchamel sauce in the microwave before making the sauce.

Nutritional value
Per serving

Calories	426
Protein	16 g
Fat	17 g
Carbohydrate	53 g
Dietary Fiber (a high source)	4 g
Calcium (a high source)	249 mg

Percent of calories from

Protein	15%
Fat	35%
Carbohydrate	50%

- Preheat oven to 375°F (190°C)
- 13- by 9-inch (3 L) baking dish, sprayed with nonstick cooking spray

12 oz	rotini or penne	375 g
4 cups	tomato meat sauce or tomato sauce	1 L

Béchamel Sauce

1/4 cup	olive oil	50 mL
1/4 cup	all-purpose flour	50 mL
4 cups	hot lactose-free milk or fortified soy milk	1 L
1	bay leaf	1
1 tsp	salt	5 mL
1/4 tsp	freshly ground black pepper	1 mL
1/4 tsp	ground nutmeg	1 mL
2 tbsp	freshly grated Parmesan cheese (optional, if tolerated)	25 mL

1. In a large pot of boiling salted water, cook pasta for 8 to 10 minutes, or until al dente (tender but firm to the bite). Drain.

2. *Prepare the Béchamel Sauce:* In a large saucepan, heat oil over medium-high heat. Gradually stir in flour and cook until flour pulls away from the side of the pan. Gradually whisk in hot milk and cook, whisking constantly, until thickened. Add bay leaf, salt, pepper and nutmeg. Cook, whisking, for 3 to 4 minutes, or until bubbly. Remove from heat.

3. Spread about 1 cup (250 mL) of the tomato sauce in bottom of prepared pan. Layer half of the pasta on top and spread with half of the remaining tomato sauce. Top with the remaining pasta, then the remaining tomato sauce. Spread béchamel sauce evenly over top layer and sprinkle with Parmesan cheese (if using).

4. Bake in preheated oven for 30 to 35 minutes, or until bubbly and browned on top. Let cool for about 10 minutes before cutting into 6 squares.

Variations

To boost calcium, add 1 to 2 cups (250 to 500 mL) blanched chopped calcium greens, such as kale or broccoli, to the lasagna, layering them between the pasta and the sauce.

To increase the protein and calcium content, add 1 cup (250 mL) chopped tofu or soybeans to the tomato sauce.

TIP

If you prefer, buy whole nutmeg and grate it with a rasp (available at cookware stores). The taste of freshly grated nutmeg is far superior to that of packaged ground nutmeg. The rasp will also work well to grate the Parmesan cheese, not to mention the zest of citrus fruits.

Garden Lasagna

Feel free to substitute any green or white vegetables you have in abundance. A combination of leek, broccoli, spinach, beans, zucchini, green pepper, cauliflower or mushrooms are all possibilities that work well to make about 14 cups (3.5 L) of chopped prepared vegetables before cooking. The packaged fresh pasta noodles are a great time-saver in this recipe, because they require no pre-cooking.

MAKES 8 SERVINGS

TIPS

For an added boost of calcium, add some braised kale with the other calcium vegetables.

Because leeks are grown mounded in sand, they often have grit or sand between the layers. To clean leeks, slice them lengthwise almost to the root and let tap water run through the various layers, removing any sand or grit.

Nutritional value
Per serving

Calories	467
Protein	20 g
Fat	15 g
Carbohydrate	67 g
Dietary Fiber (a very high source)	7 g
Calcium (a high source)	195 mg

Percent of calories from

Protein	16%
Fat	28%
Carbohydrate	56%

● Preheat oven to 350°F (180°C)
● 13- by 9-inch (3 L) baking dish, greased

1	bunch broccoli	1
1	bag (10 oz/284 g) fresh spinach	1
1	bunch (2 or 3) leeks (white part only)	1
1	head cauliflower	1
1 cup	water	250 mL
3	cloves garlic, minced	3
8 oz	mushrooms, sliced	250 g
2 tbsp	extra-virgin olive oil	25 mL
1 tsp	dried basil	5 mL
1 tsp	dried tarragon	5 mL
1/4 tsp	freshly ground black pepper	1 mL
1	package (12 oz/375 g) fresh lasagna pasta	1

Béchamel Tofu Sauce

2	packages (each 10.25 oz/290 g) silken soft tofu	2
2	eggs	2
1/4 cup	chopped fresh parsley	50 mL
2 tbsp	extra-virgin olive oil	25 mL
1 tbsp	freshly grated Parmesan cheese (optional, if tolerated)	15 mL
1 tbsp	Dijon mustard	15 mL
1/2 tsp	salt	2 mL
1/4 tsp	freshly ground black pepper	1 mL
1/4 tsp	ground nutmeg	1 mL

Seasoned Bread Crumbs

1 cup	fresh bread crumbs (preferably from Italian-style bread)	250 mL
¼ cup	chopped fresh parsley	50 mL
1 tbsp	freshly grated Parmesan cheese (optional, if tolerated)	15 mL
1 tbsp	extra-virgin olive oil	15 mL
¼ tsp	dried thyme	1 mL
¼ tsp	freshly ground black pepper	1 mL
¼ tsp	salt	1 mL

1. Trim broccoli stems and slice stalks; cut broccoli into florets. Trim spinach stems. Clean leeks and slice thinly. Cut cauliflower into florets. Rinse all vegetables under water, shaking off excess.

2. In a 24-cup (6 L) Dutch oven, bring water to a boil over high heat. In two batches, add broccoli, spinach, leeks, cauliflower, garlic, mushrooms, olive oil, basil, tarragon and pepper; reduce heat to medium and cook, covered, until florets are tender-crisp and spinach is wilted, about 5 minutes, adding more water as necessary to prevent burning. Drain and set aside.

3. *Prepare the Béchamel Tofu Sauce:* Meanwhile, using a sieve, drain tofu. In a food processor, using pulsing action, purée drained tofu, eggs, parsley, oil, cheese (if using), mustard, salt, pepper and nutmeg until smooth.

4. *Prepare the Seasoned Bread Crumbs:* In a small bowl, stir together bread crumbs, parsley, cheese (if using), oil, thyme, pepper and salt.

5. To assemble lasagna, sprinkle about 1 cup (250 mL) vegetable mixture on bottom of prepared baking dish. Cover with a layer of 2 pasta sheets. Spread half of the remaining vegetables over top. Cover with 2 more pasta sheets. Spread remaining vegetables over pasta. Top with 2 more pasta sheets. Spread Béchamel Tofu Sauce over top. Sprinkle evenly with Seasoned Bread Crumbs.

6. Bake, uncovered, in preheated oven for 25 to 30 minutes, or until heated through. Let cool for 15 minutes before cutting into squares.

TIPS

Clean mushrooms with a damp cloth. Do not immerse them in water — they soak up water like a sponge.

Store fresh mushrooms in the refrigerator for up to 1 week in a paper bag rather than in plastic, where they are too moist and become slimy.

Look for fresh lasagna noodles (sheets) in the refrigerated deli section of the grocery store.

To get ¼ cup (50 mL) chopped fresh parsley, you will need about one small bunch. Any leftover parsley may be chopped and frozen in a freezer container.

Florentine Lasagna

This version is so bursting with flavor that no one will ever miss the usual quantities of cheese in the traditional dish. Fresh pasta sheets speed up preparation.

MAKES 8 SERVINGS

TIP

If you prefer, you can make the Béchamel Tofu Sauce in the Garden Lasagna (see recipe, page 120) to replace this béchamel sauce.

- Preheat oven to 350°F (180°C).
- 13- by 9-inch (3 L) baking dish, greased or sprayed with nonstick baking spray

1 lb	lean ground beef	500 g
2	cloves garlic, chopped	2
1	onion, chopped	1
1/2	green bell pepper, chopped	1/2
8 oz	mushrooms, sliced	250 g
2 tsp	dried basil	10 mL
1	can (28 oz/796 mL) tomatoes	1
1	can (5 1/2 oz/156 mL) tomato paste	1
1 tsp	liquid honey	5 mL
1 tsp	salt	5 mL
1/4 tsp	freshly ground black pepper	1 mL
1	package (12 oz/375 g) fresh lasagna pasta	1

Béchamel Sauce

1/4 cup	all-purpose flour	50 mL
2 tbsp	vegetable oil	25 mL
1 1/2 cups	lactose-free milk	375 mL
1	bay leaf	1
1 tbsp	freshly grated Parmesan cheese (optional, if tolerated)	15 mL
1/4 tsp	salt	1 mL
Pinch	freshly ground black pepper	Pinch
Pinch	ground nutmeg	Pinch

Nutritional value
Per serving

Calories	391
Protein	19 g
Fat	18 g
Carbohydrate	40 g
Dietary Fiber (a high source)	5 g
Calcium (a source)	143 mg

Percent of calories from

Protein	19%
Fat	41%
Carbohydrate	40%

Bread Crumb Topping

½ cup	fine dry bread crumbs	125 mL
2 tbsp	chopped fresh parsley	25 mL
2 tbsp	extra-virgin olive oil	25 mL
1 tbsp	freshly grated Parmesan cheese (optional, if tolerated)	15 mL

1. In a Dutch oven or large saucepan, over medium-high heat, brown beef with garlic and onion until onion is softened, about 5 minutes. Stir in green pepper, mushrooms and basil; cook until mushrooms release liquid, about 5 minutes. Stir in tomatoes and tomato paste, breaking up tomatoes; cook for 10 minutes. Season with honey, salt and pepper.

2. *Prepare the Béchamel Sauce:* In a large heavy saucepan, stir together flour and oil; cook, stirring, over medium heat until pale brown. Gradually stir in milk and bay leaf; cook, stirring, for 8 to 10 minutes, or until thickened and smooth. Stir in cheese (if using), salt, pepper and nutmeg. Discard bay leaf.

3. *Prepare the Bread Crumb Topping:* In a small bowl, stir together bread crumbs, parsley, oil and cheese (if using).

4. To assemble lasagna, spread about 2 cups (500 mL) meat sauce on bottom of prepared baking dish. Arrange 2 sheets of pasta over sauce. Spread half of the remaining sauce over pasta. Top with 2 more sheets. Spread remaining sauce over pasta. Top with 2 more sheets of pasta. Spread béchamel sauce over top. Sprinkle with bread crumb topping.

5. Bake in preheated oven for 30 to 35 minutes, or until heated through. Let stand for 15 minutes before cutting into squares.

MAKE AHEAD

Béchamel sauce can be stored in an airtight container in the freezer for up to 2 months. Thaw over low heat, whisking, to bring back the smooth texture. Use either as a pasta sauce or for the lasagna. Lasagna can be covered and stored in the refrigerator for up to 12 hours. Reheat in a preheated 350°F (180°C) oven for 35 to 40 minutes, or until heated through.

Margherita Pizza

Although pizza with oodles of gooey cheese is off-limits to the lactose intolerant, many can digest small quantities of hard aged cheeses, such as Parmesan.

MAKES ONE 12-INCH (30 CM) PIZZA

TIPS

Hard aged cheese, such as Parmesan, is often tolerated by those who are lactose intolerant. However, this will vary on an individual basis. If you cannot tolerate Parmesan, try lactose-free Parmesan cheese, available at many supermarkets and health food stores.

If fresh basil is not available, use 2 tbsp (25 mL) dried.

- ● Preheat oven to 425°F (220°C)
- ● 12-inch (30 cm) pizza pan

1	12-inch (30 cm) pre-baked pizza shell	1
2 tbsp	olive oil, divided	25 mL
2	large ripe tomatoes, thinly sliced	2
1 cup	freshly grated Parmesan cheese (see tip, at left)	250 mL
¼ cup	sliced fresh basil	50 mL
¼ tsp	freshly ground black pepper	1 mL

1. Place pizza shell in pan and brush with 1 tbsp (15 mL) of the oil. Arrange tomato slices in a single layer on pizza shell. Drizzle with the remaining oil. Sprinkle evenly with cheese, basil and pepper.

2. Bake in preheated oven for 10 to 15 minutes, or until cheese is beginning to melt. Cut into 6 wedges and serve.

Nutritional value
Per serving (⅙th of pizza)

Calories	178
Protein	9 g
Fat	11 g
Carbohydrate	13 g
Dietary Fiber	1 g
Calcium (a high source)	241 mg

Percent of calories from

Protein	19%
Fat	52%
Carbohydrate	29%

Pesto Pizza

Homemade Parsley Pesto is my favorite emergency staple. I try to have a jar in the freezer at all times. It's great for appetizers (Sun-Dried Tomato and Parsley Pesto Dip, page 26), it makes a wonderful pasta topping, and it never fails to please pizza lovers. With a bare sprinkling of cheese, it's lip-smacking good!

MAKES ONE 12-INCH (30 CM) PIZZA

TIP

Kitchen scissors work well to cut pizza into neat wedges.

● *Preheat oven to 425°F (220°C)*
● *Baking sheet*

½ cup	Parsley Pesto (see recipe, page 27)	125 mL
1	12-inch (30 cm) pre-baked pizza shell	1
2	large tomatoes, sliced	2
1 cup	freshly grated Parmesan cheese (optional, if tolerated)	250 mL

1. Spread pesto on pizza shell. Arrange sliced tomatoes across surface. Place on baking sheet.

2. Bake in preheated oven for 20 to 25 minutes, or until heated through. Sprinkle evenly with cheese (if using). Cut into 6 wedges and serve hot or at room temperature.

Nutritional value
Per serving (⅙th of pizza)

Calories	402
Protein	15 g
Fat	19 g
Carbohydrate	39 g
Dietary Fiber (a source)	2 g
Calcium (a very high source)	341 mg

Percent of calories from

Protein	17%
Fat	40%
Carbohydrate	43%

Bruschetta Pizza

For added protein and calcium, sprinkle pizza with the marinated crumbled tofu. Serve piping hot or at room temperature for packed lunches.

MAKES ONE 12-INCH (30 CM) PIZZA

TIP

If you are running short on time, use a purchased 12-inch (30 cm) pizza shell. Brush with olive oil, sprinkle with rosemary and toppings and bake at 425°F (220°C) for 20 to 25 minutes, or until heated through. Pizza dough is available in the deli refrigerator counters of the supermarket.

Nutritional value
Per serving (¹⁄₆th of pizza)

Calories	317
Protein	10 g
Fat	12 g
Carbohydrate	43 g
Dietary Fiber (a source)	2 g
Calcium	34 mg

Percent of calories from

Protein	13%
Fat	33%
Carbohydrate	54%

● *Preheat oven to 450°F (230°C)*
● *12-inch (30 cm) pizza pan, greased or sprayed with nonstick baking spray*

Marinated Tofu (optional)

6 oz	extra-firm tofu, crumbled	175 g
1 tbsp	extra-virgin olive oil	15 mL
2 tsp	balsamic vinegar	10 mL
1 tsp	dried rosemary	5 mL

Crust

1	package (12 oz/375 g) pizza dough	1
2 tsp	extra-virgin olive oil	10 mL
½ tsp	dried rosemary	2 mL

Topping

2	large tomatoes, chopped (2 cups/500 mL)	2
2	cloves garlic, minced	2
½ cup	chopped red onion	125 mL
¼ cup	chopped fresh parsley	50 mL
2 tbsp	extra-virgin olive oil	25 mL
2 tsp	dried basil	10 mL
½ tsp	salt	2 mL

Freshly grated Parmesan cheese (optional, if tolerated)

1. *Prepare the Marinated Tofu (if using):* In a small bowl, combine tofu, oil, vinegar and rosemary. Let stand for about 10 minutes.

2. *Meanwhile, prepare the crust:* Roll dough out on a floured surface to fit prepared pizza pan. Brush with oil and sprinkle with rosemary. Bake in preheated oven until pale brown, about 5 minutes.

3. *Meanwhile, prepare the topping:* Combine tomatoes, garlic, onion, parsley, oil, basil and salt.

4. Sprinkle partially baked crust evenly with topping and marinated tofu (if using). Bake until golden brown on bottom, about 20 minutes. Remove from oven and sprinkle with cheese (if using). Cut into 6 wedges and serve hot or at room temperature.

TIP

Balsamic vinegar is an aged vinegar. Like a good wine, the older the vinegar, the more mellow the taste. You don't need to buy the most expensive vinegar, but try to buy it from a store where knowledgeable staff can answer questions or perhaps give you a taste before you buy.

Roasted Ratatouille Pizza

All the flavors of a classic ratatouille — eggplant, zucchini, peppers, garlic and tomatoes — combine in this roasted version as a pizza topping.

MAKES ONE 12-INCH (30 CM) PIZZA

TIPS

There are a variety of eggplants on the market. Whatever type you choose, make sure the skin is shiny and free of bruises or blemishes, and the eggplant is firm to the touch. Choose one that is small in size — it will be sweeter.

For a dramatic presentation, use tri-colored peppers (red, yellow and orange) and use half a green zucchini and half a yellow summer squash.

Nutritional value
Per serving (1/6th of pizza)

Calories	238
Protein	7 g
Fat	7 g
Carbohydrate	37 g
Dietary Fiber (a high source)	4 g
Calcium	35 mg

Percent of calories from

Protein	12%
Fat	26%
Carbohydrate	62%

● *Preheat broiler*
● *Baking sheet*

8	mushrooms, halved	8
2	cloves garlic, minced	2
1	small eggplant, sliced in 1/2-inch (1 cm) rounds	1
1	small zucchini, sliced	1
1/2	red bell pepper, halved	1/2
1/2	red onion, sliced	1/2
2 tbsp	extra-virgin olive oil	25 mL
1	12-inch (30 cm) baked pizza shell	1
1 tbsp	freshly grated Parmesan cheese (optional, if tolerated)	15 mL
1 tbsp	balsamic vinegar	15 mL
1 tsp	dried basil	5 mL
1 tsp	dried rosemary	5 mL
1 tsp	dried thyme	5 mL
	Coarse salt and freshly ground black pepper	

1. Arrange mushrooms, garlic, eggplant, zucchini, red pepper (cut side down) and red onion on baking sheet. Using pastry brush, paint lightly with oil. Broil for 2 to 3 minutes, or until browned and lightly charred. Remove all vegetables except pepper. Continue broiling pepper until blackened.

2. Meanwhile, arrange vegetables on pizza shell.

3. Place charred pepper in a plastic container with lid. Let stand for 10 minutes. Peel and slice; arrange evenly over pizza. Preheat oven to 425°F (220°C).

4. Sprinkle pizza with cheese (if using), balsamic vinegar, basil, rosemary, thyme and salt and pepper to taste.

5. Place on baking sheet and bake for 15 to 20 minutes, or until heated through. Cut into 6 wedges and serve hot or at room temperature.

TIP

The best Parmesan cheese is Parmigiano Reggiano, which has a sweet, nutty taste quite different from the strong salty taste of the grated cheese sold in plastic containers or canisters. However, for this recipe, the less expensive version is fine — you're using such a small quantity, you can use the more powerful flavor kick.

Four Onion Pizza with Rosemary

Onions and their relatives, shallots, garlic and leeks, become as sweet as candy when slowly sautéed. Sprinkle with some fresh or dried herbs, and you have a mouth-watering pizza.

MAKES ONE 12-INCH (30 CM) PIZZA

TIP

When you sprinkle cheese on pizza as it comes out of the oven, it melts nicely without being tough and chewy, as it would have been if baked in the oven.

- Preheat oven to 450°F (230°C)
- 12-inch (30 cm) pizza pan, greased or sprayed with nonstick baking spray

2 tbsp	extra-virgin olive oil	25 mL
2	onions, sliced	2
2	shallots, chopped	2
2	cloves garlic, minced	2
1	leek (white part only), thinly sliced	1
1 tsp	dried rosemary	5 mL
1	package (12 oz/375 g) pizza dough	1
1 cup	freshly grated Parmesan or Asiago cheese (optional, if tolerated)	250 mL

1. In a heavy saucepan, heat oil over medium heat. Cook onions, shallots, garlic, leek and rosemary, covered, for 10 to 12 minutes, or until softened.

2. Meanwhile, on a floured surface, roll out dough to fit prepared pizza pan. Bake in preheated oven for 5 to 8 minutes, or until pale brown.

3. Spread onion mixture over dough and bake for 20 to 25 minutes, or until golden brown on bottom. Remove from oven and sprinkle with cheese (if using). Cut into 6 wedges and serve hot or at room temperature.

Nutritional value
Per serving (¹/₆th of pizza)

Calories	296
Protein	13 g
Fat	11 g
Carbohydrate	35 g
Dietary Fiber (a source)	2 g
Calcium (a high source)	252 mg

Percent of calories from

Protein	18%
Fat	35%
Carbohydrate	47%

Main Courses

Naturally, there is no lactose in poultry, fish or meat when it is baked or grilled simply with herbs and a squeeze of lemon. However, these foods lend themselves to magnificent cream-based sauces that cause problems for lactose-intolerant people. The dishes here include basic lactose-free sauces rich in flavor to replace their cream-based cousins.

Vegetarian Chili 132

Chicken Chili 133

Chicken without Bother 134

Chicken Divan 135

Chicken Pot Pie with Leeks
and Mushrooms 136

Creamy Chicken Curry 138

Shepherd's Pie 140

Chicken Fingers with Creamy
Dipping Sauce 142

Turkey Sausages 143

Herb-Roasted Turkey 144

Tuna Primavera 145

Fish Fingers 146

Fisherman's Pie 148

Easy Salmon Pie 150

Grilled Salmon 152

Salmon Mousse 153

Salmon Loaf 154

Burgers with the Works 155

Veal and Mushrooms 156

Beef Stroganoff 158

Vegetarian Chili

One of my favorite recipes, this is sure to fight off the winter blahs! Serve it over rice or with Tortilla Chips (see recipe, page 35).

(see recipe, page 35)

MAKES 6 SERVINGS

TIP

All beans contain some calcium, but soybeans contain the most.

MAKE AHEAD

Ladle into an airtight container and store in the refrigerator for up to 2 days or in the freezer for up to 1 month.

Nutritional value
Per serving

Calories	504
Protein	33 g
Fat	16 g
Carbohydrate	65 g
Dietary Fiber (a very high source)	17 g
Calcium (a high source)	257 mg

Percent of calories from

Protein	25%
Fat	27%
Carbohydrate	49%

2 tbsp	vegetable oil	25 mL
2	cloves garlic, minced	2
1	large onion, chopped	1
2 tsp	chili powder	10 mL
1 tsp	ground cumin	5 mL
1 tsp	dried oregano	5 mL
1	can (28 oz/796 mL) diced tomatoes	1
1	can (19 oz/540 mL) soybeans, rinsed and drained	1
1	can (19 oz/540 mL) white or red kidney beans	1
1	can (19 oz/540 mL) chickpeas	1
1	green bell pepper, coarsely chopped	1
1 tbsp	cider vinegar	15 mL
1/2 tsp	salt	2 mL
1/2 tsp	ground cinnamon	2 mL
1/4 tsp	freshly ground black pepper	1 mL
1/4 cup	chopped fresh cilantro	50 mL

1. In a large saucepan, heat oil over medium-high heat. Cook garlic and onion, covered, until softened, about 5 minutes. Stir in chili powder, cumin and oregano; cook, stirring, for 2 minutes. Stir in tomatoes with juice, soybeans, kidney beans, chickpeas, green pepper, vinegar, salt, cinnamon and pepper. Bring to a boil; reduce heat to medium-low and simmer, uncovered, for 20 minutes to allow flavors to blend.

2. Just before serving, stir in cilantro. Taste and adjust seasoning as desired with salt and pepper.

Variations

For a splash of color, add 1 cup (250 mL) frozen corn.

For meat eaters, add 1 lb (500 g) cooked lean ground beef or chicken.

Chicken Chili

An old-fashioned favorite with a new face, this version has extra calcium with the addition of soybeans.

MAKES 4 SERVINGS

MAKE AHEAD

Ladle chili into airtight containers and store in the refrigerator for up to 2 days or in the freezer for up to 3 months. Be sure to date and label freezer containers.

1 lb	lean ground chicken	500 g
1	large onion, chopped	1
1	clove garlic, minced	1
1	can (28 oz/796 mL) diced tomatoes	1
1	can (19 oz/540 mL) soybeans, rinsed and drained	1
1 tbsp	chili powder	15 mL
½ tsp	dried oregano	2 mL
½ tsp	ground cumin	2 mL
½ tsp	salt	2 mL
¼ tsp	freshly ground black pepper	1 mL
	Rice or tortillas	

1. In a large saucepan, over medium heat, cook chicken, onion and garlic, breaking meat up, for 5 to 7 minutes, or until chicken is no longer pink. Stir in tomatoes with juice, soybeans, chili powder, oregano, cumin, salt and pepper. Cook, stirring frequently, for about 10 minutes to allow flavors to blend.

2. Meanwhile, cook rice as per package instructions (or wrap tortillas in foil and heat in a 350°F/180°C oven for about 10 minutes).

3. Serve chili over rice or in a warmed tortilla.

Variation

If you wish, substitute chickpeas or kidney beans for soybeans, but remember that they contain less calcium.

Nutritional value
Per serving

Calories	512
Protein	42 g
Fat	22 g
Carbohydrate	40 g
Dietary Fiber (a high source)	5 g
Calcium (a high source)	257 mg

Percent of calories from

Protein	32%
Fat	38%
Carbohydrate	30%

Chicken without Bother

This is the lazy cook's recipe for preparing succulent, tender chicken in a tasty broth for any of those popular creamy casseroles, pasta dishes and salads, or simply to eat on its own. The leftover stock is invaluable for creating a mouth-watering Basic Béchamel Sauce for Chicken Dishes (see recipe, page 243). Once cooled, the chicken fat can easily be skimmed from the stock. A little chicken fat can then be used for added flavor in the Basic Béchamel Sauce.

MAKES ABOUT 3 CUPS (750 ML) CHICKEN AND 1 CUP (250 ML) CHICKEN STOCK

TIP

Free-range and air-chilled chickens will have more flavor than the more common supermarket variety.

MAKE AHEAD

Chicken and chicken stock can be stored in the refrigerator for up to 2 days or in the freezer for up to 2 months.

Nutritional value
Per serving (1 cup/250 mL chicken)

Calories	478
Protein	68 g
Fat	18 g
Carbohydrate	1 g
Dietary Fiber	0 g
Calcium	46 mg

Percent of calories from

Protein	59%
Fat	34%
Carbohydrate	1%

- Preheat oven to 375°F (190°C)
- 11- by 7-inch (2 L) baking dish, greased or sprayed with nonstick baking spray

1	chicken (3 lbs/1.5 kg) or chicken pieces	1
1 cup	chicken stock	250 mL
1/2 cup	white wine	125 mL
1/2 tsp	dried thyme	2 mL
1/2 tsp	dried tarragon	2 mL
1	bay leaf	1

1. Rinse and pat chicken dry. Arrange in prepared baking dish.

2. In a measuring cup, stir together chicken stock, wine, thyme, tarragon and bay leaf; pour over chicken. Cover loosely with foil.

3. Bake in preheated oven for 1 1/2 to 2 hours, or until drumsticks wiggle easily and meat thermometer inserted in thickest part of thigh registers 185°F (85°C).

4. When chicken is cool enough to handle, remove meat from carcass; discard bones and skin. Pour remaining chicken stock mixture into an airtight container and refrigerate. Chicken fat can be removed from stock once chilled. Cover chicken and refrigerate until ready to use in a recipe.

Chicken Divan

A comforting dish suitable for guests but easy enough for a weekday meal, this can be made up to a day ahead, covered and refrigerated until ready to reheat. Serve with a salad and rice.

MAKES 4 SERVINGS

TIP

Recipe doubles easily to serve 8, but requires a 13- by 9-inch (3 L) baking dish.

- Preheat oven to 350°F (180°C)
- 8-inch (2 L) square baking dish, greased

1	bunch broccoli	1
3 cups	cooked chicken pieces (see Chicken without Bother, opposite)	750 mL
2 cups	Basic Béchamel Sauce for Chicken Dishes (see recipe, page 243)	500 mL

Bread Crumb Topping

½ cup	fine dry bread crumbs	125 mL
2 tbsp	extra-virgin olive oil	25 mL
2 tbsp	freshly grated Parmesan cheese (optional, if tolerated)	25 mL

1. In a large saucepan, bring about 1 inch (2.5 cm) water to a boil over high heat.

2. Meanwhile, cut off tough part of broccoli stems; slice lengthwise into florets with stem attached. Cook in saucepan of boiling water, uncovered, until tender-crisp, about 3 minutes. Drain and cool.

3. Arrange broccoli in a single layer in prepared baking dish. Arrange chicken over broccoli. Spread Basic Béchamel Sauce over chicken.

4. *Prepare the Bread Crumb Topping:* In a small bowl, stir together bread crumbs, oil and cheese (if using) until well blended. Sprinkle evenly over sauce.

5. Bake in preheated oven, uncovered, for 35 to 40 minutes, or until heated through and bread crumbs are browned.

Nutritional value
Per serving

Calories	390
Protein	26 g
Fat	21 g
Carbohydrate	23 g
Dietary Fiber (a high source)	4 g
Calcium (a high source)	199 mg

Percent of calories from

Protein	27%
Fat	48%
Carbohydrate	23%

Chicken Pot Pie with Leeks and Mushrooms

This lactose-free treat can be made from soy milk or lactose-free milk instead of cream. Serve with Nice 'n' Nutty Slaw (see recipe, page 102) and crusty bread.

MAKES 4 SERVINGS

TIPS

Because leeks are grown mounded in sand, they often have grit or sand between the layers. To clean leeks, slice them lengthwise almost to the root and let tap water run through the various layers, removing any sand or grit.

Clean mushrooms with a damp cloth. Do not immerse them in water — they soak up water like a sponge.

Nutritional value
Per serving

Calories	577
Protein	26 g
Fat	32 g
Carbohydrate	45 g
Dietary Fiber (a very high source)	6 g
Calcium (a source)	148 mg

Percent of calories from

Protein	18%
Fat	49%
Carbohydrate	31%

- Preheat oven to 425°F (220°C)
- 8-cup (2 L) baking dish, greased or sprayed with nonstick baking spray

Filling

1 tbsp	chicken fat or vegetable oil	15 mL
8 oz	mushrooms, sliced	250 g
2 cups	sliced leeks	500 mL
2 cups	julienned carrots	500 mL
1 cup	sliced celery	250 mL
3 cups	cooked chicken pieces (see Chicken without Bother, page 134)	750 mL
2 cups	Basic Béchamel Sauce for Chicken Dishes (see recipe, page 243)	500 mL
½ cup	chicken stock (store-bought or see recipe, page 68)	125 mL
½ tsp	dried thyme	2 mL

Pastry

1 cup	all-purpose flour	250 mL
¼ tsp	salt	1 mL
⅓ cup	shortening	75 mL
3 tbsp	cold water	50 mL

1. *Prepare the filling:* In large saucepan, melt chicken fat over medium heat. Cook mushrooms, leeks, carrots and celery for 4 to 5 minutes, or until tender. Stir in chicken, Basic Béchamel Sauce, stock and thyme. Spoon into prepared baking dish.

2. *Prepare the pastry:* In a medium bowl, stir together flour and salt. Using a pastry blender or 2 knives, cut in shortening until mixture resembles fine crumbs. Stir in water with a fork and form into a ball. Roll out between 2 sheets of waxed paper and fit on top of chicken mixture. Cut vents in pastry.

3. Bake in preheated oven for 25 to 30 minutes, or until crust is pale brown.

TIPS

Rolling out pastry is easy, with no mess, when you put the pastry between 2 sheets of waxed paper and roll away from your body. Roll first in one direction, then turn waxed paper and roll again to make a circular shape.

If you are pastry challenged or simply short on time, buy a frozen prepared pie shell to replace the homemade pastry.

Creamy Chicken Curry

A dish described as "creamy" doesn't have to be taboo. This recipe uses coconut milk and yogurt to create the creamy consistency.

MAKES 6 SERVINGS

TIPS

An authentic curry is not just one spice but a mixture of fresh spices fried together before the other ingredients are added.

In Indian cooking, chili pepper refers to a hot red pepper similar to cayenne pepper. It can be found in Indian markets. If you like hot dishes, simply add more chili pepper.

Nutritional value
Per serving

Calories	620
Protein	53 g
Fat	37 g
Carbohydrate	19 g
Dietary Fiber (a source)	2 g
Calcium (a source)	103 mg

Percent of calories from

Protein	34%
Fat	54%
Carbohydrate	12%

- Preheat oven to 350°F (180°C)
- Baking sheet

2 tbsp	vegetable oil	25 mL
2	cloves garlic, minced	2
1	large onion, chopped	1
1	cinnamon stick	1
1 tbsp	minced gingerroot	15 mL
1 tsp	coriander seeds	5 mL
½ tsp	ground turmeric	2 mL
¼ tsp	chili pepper (see tip, at left)	2 mL
¼ tsp	ground cloves	1 mL
2½ lbs	boneless skinless chicken thighs	1.25 kg
1 cup	coconut milk	250 mL
1 cup	plain yogurt (see tip, at right)	250 mL
½ cup	cashews	125 mL
½ cup	chopped dried apricots	125 mL
¼ cup	chopped fresh cilantro	50 mL

1. In a large saucepan, heat oil over medium heat. Cook garlic, onion, cinnamon stick, ginger, coriander seeds, turmeric, chili pepper and cloves, stirring frequently, until onion is softened, about 5 minutes. Add chicken and brown in the spicy oil mixture.

2. Stir in coconut milk and yogurt. Add up to 1 cup (250 mL) water if chicken mixture is too dry. Increase heat to medium-high and bring to a boil; reduce heat to low, cover and simmer, stirring occasionally, until chicken reaches an internal temperature of 170°F (75°C) and juices run clear, about 30 minutes.

3. Meanwhile, place cashews on baking sheet and toast in preheated oven for 10 to 15 minutes, or until fragrant and pale brown.

4. Serve chicken garnished with toasted cashews, apricots and cilantro.

TIP

If you cannot tolerate yogurt, omit and add ½ cup (125 mL) coconut milk and ½ cup (125 mL) water. Omit the additional water in the recipe.

Shepherd's Pie

This old-timer gets a makeover with a sweet potato topping and a chicken or turkey filling.

MAKES 4 SERVINGS

TIPS

Although sweet potatoes contain calcium, it is unavailable to us because it contains oxalic acid, which makes the absorption of calcium difficult.

Clean mushrooms with a damp cloth. Do not immerse them in water — they soak up water like a sponge.

Store fresh mushrooms in the refrigerator for up to 1 week in a paper bag rather than in plastic, where they are too moist and become slimy.

Nutritional value
Per serving

Calories	513
Protein	33 g
Fat	15 g
Carbohydrate	62 g
Dietary Fiber (a very high source)	9 g
Calcium (a high source)	204 mg

Percent of calories from

Protein	25%
Fat	25%
Carbohydrate	50%

- Preheat oven to 350°F (180°C)
- 8-cup (2 L) baking dish

Topping

2½ lbs	sweet potatoes, peeled and quartered	1.25 kg
½ cup	lactose-free milk or fortified soy milk	125 mL
½ tsp	salt	2 mL
¼ tsp	freshly ground black pepper	1 mL

Filling

1 lb	lean ground chicken or turkey	500 g
2	cloves garlic, minced	2
1	onion, chopped	1
1	stalk celery, sliced	1
8 oz	mushrooms, sliced	250 g
½ tsp	salt	2 mL
¼ tsp	freshly ground black pepper	1 mL
¼ tsp	dried thyme	1 mL
2 tbsp	minced fresh parsley	25 mL
1 tbsp	all-purpose flour	15 mL
½ cup	lactose-free milk or fortified soy milk	125 mL

1. *Prepare the topping:* Place sweet potatoes in a large saucepan and add enough cold water to cover. Bring to a boil over high heat; reduce heat to medium, cover and cook for 12 to 15 minutes, or until tender when pierced with the tip of a knife. Drain and mash with milk, salt and pepper.

2. *Meanwhile, prepare the filling:* In another large saucepan, over medium-high heat, cook chicken, stirring to break up, for 5 to 7 minutes, or until no longer pink. Add garlic, onion, celery, mushrooms, salt, pepper and thyme. Cover and cook for 10 minutes, until vegetables are softened. Stir in parsley and flour Gradually stir in milk.

3. Spoon chicken mixture into baking dish. Spoon mashed potatoes on top, making decorative swirls. Bake in preheated oven for 40 to 45 minutes, or until heated through.

Variations

Substitute ground beef for the chicken or turkey.

Substitute white potatoes for the sweet potatoes.

TIP

If you prefer, substitute 1 tsp (5 mL) chopped fresh thyme for the dried thyme.

MAKE AHEAD

Cover and store in the refrigerator for up to 1 day. Reheat in a 350°F (180°C) oven for 40 to 45 minutes, or until bubbly.

Chicken Fingers with Creamy Dipping Sauce

Convenience foods such as chicken fingers are often coated in a breading mixture that contains lactose. This easy recipe eliminates the problem.

MAKES 4 SERVINGS

TIP

Sesame seeds contain calcium. Wherever possible, include them in recipes for their added crunch, taste and calcium.

- Preheat oven to 425°F (220°C)
- Baking sheet, lined with parchment paper

1 lb	boneless skinless chicken breast	500 g
1	egg	1
½ cup	fine dry bread crumbs	125 mL
¼ cup	sesame seeds	50 mL
½ tsp	dried thyme	2 mL
	Creamy Veggie Dip (see recipe, page 24)	

1. Using a sharp knife, cut chicken breasts crosswise into 2- by ½-inch (5 by 1 cm) fingers.

2. In a shallow bowl, whisk together egg and 1 tbsp (15 mL) water.

3. In a separate shallow bowl, stir together bread crumbs, sesame seeds and thyme.

4. Dip chicken in egg mixture, turning to coat, then in bread crumb mixture, turning to coat all sides. Arrange on prepared baking sheet.

5. Bake in preheated oven for 20 to 25 minutes, or until no longer pink inside.

6. Serve immediately with Creamy Veggie Dip.

Nutritional value
Per serving (without dip)

Calories	251
Protein	31 g
Fat	8 g
Carbohydrate	12 g
Dietary Fiber	1 g
Calcium (a source)	134 mg

Percent of calories from

Protein	50%
Fat	30%
Carbohydrate	20%

Turkey Sausages

Commercial sausages and wieners are hidden sources of lactose because skim milk powder is often used as a filler. Not these. If you like sausages, you'll love this lactose-free version. They are low in fat, a snap to make, and they taste great!

MAKES 4 SERVINGS

TIP

Serve in a sesame seed roll with Dijon mustard and pickles.

1 lb	ground turkey	500 g
1	clove garlic, crushed	1
1/4 cup	dry bread crumbs	50 mL
1/2 tsp	salt	2 mL
1/2 tsp	powdered sage	2 mL
1/4 tsp	ground nutmeg	1 mL
1/4 tsp	freshly ground black pepper	1 mL

1. In a medium bowl, combine turkey, garlic, bread crumbs, salt, sage, nutmeg and pepper until spices are evenly distributed. Shape into wiener, meatball or patty shapes.

2. Cook in a nonstick skillet over medium-high heat for about 15 minutes, turning, until brown on all sides and cooked through.

Nutritional value
Per serving

Calories	167
Protein	16 g
Fat	9 g
Carbohydrate	5 g
Dietary Fiber	0 g
Calcium	29 mg

Percent of calories from

Protein	39%
Fat	49%
Carbohydrate	12%

Herb-Roasted Turkey

Once you have prepared your turkey using this no-fuss method on the barbecue, you are a convert for life! It cooks in double-quick time and leaves your oven free for all the vegetable casseroles.

MAKES ABOUT 12 SERVINGS

TIPS

Do not use a pre-basted turkey for this method. The added oil will flare up on the barbecue.

Spread liquid dishwasher detergent on the outside of roasting pan for easy cleanup, or use a disposable foil pan.

● *Preheat barbecue to medium-high*
● *Roasting pan*

1	fresh turkey (12 to 16 lbs/5.5 to 7.25 kg)	1
1	onion	1
1	stalk celery	1
2 tbsp	freshly squeezed lemon juice	25 mL
2 tbsp	olive oil	25 mL
2 tsp	dried thyme	10 mL
½ tsp	dried rosemary	2 mL
2 to 3 cups	water	500 to 750 mL

1. Remove neck and giblets from turkey. Rinse turkey under cold water and pat dry with paper towels. Tuck wings under back. Place on rack in pan.

2. Place onion and celery in cavity. Squeeze lemon juice on outside of bird. Sprinkle evenly with oil, thyme and rosemary. Pour in water. Cover bird with 2 layers of foil.

3. Place on barbecue grill; close lid. Cook, replenishing water if necessary, for 2 to 2½ hours, or until meat thermometer inserted in thickest part of thigh registers 180°F (82°C). Remove from pan and let stand, covered, for 15 minutes before carving.

Nutritional value
Per serving

Calories	646
Protein	105 g
Fat	21 g
Carbohydrate	2 g
Dietary Fiber	0 g
Calcium (a source)	103 mg

Percent of calories from

Protein	68%
Fat	31%
Carbohydrate	1%

Tuna Primavera

Remember that much-loved tuna casserole? Here's a revamped version, using soy milk to make a speedy sauce for noodles or rice the whole family can enjoy.

MAKES ABOUT 3 CUPS (750 ML)

TIP

Cook rice or pasta according to package directions. Allow 2 cups (500 mL) uncooked parboiled rice for 4 servings and 12 oz to 1 lb (375 to 500 g) pasta for 4 servings.

1 tbsp	vegetable oil	15 mL
1	stalk celery, chopped	1
1	small onion, chopped	1
1	clove garlic, minced	1
1/3	chopped red or green bell pepper	75 mL
8 oz	mushrooms, sliced	250 g
1 tbsp	all-purpose flour	15 mL
1 1/2 cups	fortified soy milk or lactose-free milk	375 mL
1	can (6.5 oz/184 g) tuna packed in water, drained	1
1 tbsp	ketchup	15 mL
1 tsp	Worcestershire sauce	5 mL
1/2 tsp	salt	2 mL
	Cooked rice or pasta	
1/4 cup	chopped fresh parsley	50 mL

1. In a large saucepan, heat oil over medium heat; cook celery, onion, garlic, red pepper and mushrooms, covered, for 8 to 10 minutes, or until onions are softened. Sprinkle with flour, stirring to combine. Gradually stir in soy milk; cook, stirring, until thickened. Stir in tuna, ketchup, Worcestershire sauce and salt until well combined.

2. Spoon over rice or pasta and sprinkle with parsley.

Variation

Substitute canned salmon, with crushed bones, for the tuna. Canned salmon is an excellent source of vitamin D and calcium.

Nutritional value
Per serving (3/4 cup/175 mL)

Calories	160
Protein	17 g
Fat	6 g
Carbohydrate	11 g
Dietary Fiber (a source)	3 g
Calcium	33 mg

Percent of calories from

Protein	42%
Fat	31%
Carbohydrate	27%

Fish Fingers

Breading for fish and chicken in the popular frozen food section of the supermarket is a hidden source of lactose (milk powder in the bread crumbs), which can cause problems for those with lactose intolerance. This recipe makes everyone happy.

MAKES 4 SERVINGS

TIPS

To make dry bread crumbs, toast bread, let it cool, then process it to fine crumbs in a blender or processor. You'll likely need two slices for ½ cup (125 mL) of crumbs.

The method for fresh fillets is different from that for frozen fillets because bread crumbs will stick to fresh fillets but not frozen ones.

Nutritional value
Per serving

Calories	222
Protein	18 g
Fat	12 g
Carbohydrate	10 g
Dietary Fiber	1 g
Calcium	31 mg

Percent of calories from

Protein	33%
Fat	49%
Carbohydrate	18%

- Preheat oven to 450°F (230°C)
- 13- by 9-inch (3 L) baking dish, greased

Breading

½ cup	dry bread crumbs (see tip, at left)	125 mL
¼ tsp	salt	1 mL
¼ tsp	paprika	1 mL
¼ tsp	dried thyme	1 mL
¼ tsp	granulated sugar	1 mL
¼ tsp	freshly ground black pepper	1 mL
2 tbsp	vegetable oil	25 mL
1	package (14 oz/400 g) individually frozen fish fillets (sole, haddock or cod), thawed (or use fresh)	1
1 tbsp	vegetable oil	15 mL

1. *Prepare the breading:* In a small bowl, stir together bread crumbs, salt, paprika, thyme, sugar and pepper. Stir in oil.
2. Cut each fillet in half lengthwise to make a long, fat "finger."

3. Brush frozen fillets with oil, arrange in a single layer in prepared baking dish and sprinkle breading evenly over fillets. (If using fresh fillets, brush lightly with oil and dip into bread crumbs to coat on each side. Arrange in a single layer in baking dish.)

4. Bake in preheated oven for 10 to 15 minutes, or until fish flakes easily when tested with a fork.

Variation

Chicken Fingers: Substitute fresh chicken strips for fish and bake at 375°F (190°C) for 30 to 35 minutes, or until no longer pink inside.

TIP

Fish fingers are delicious with Green Sauce (see recipe, page 245).

Fisherman's Pie

Children are guaranteed to like this soothing dish, with a mashed potato crust and a well-seasoned filling.

MAKES 4 SERVINGS

TIPS

To increase the calcium content, substitute 1 stalk of coarsely chopped bok choy for the celery. Serve with Nice 'n' Nutty Slaw (see recipe, page 102).

Clean mushrooms with a damp cloth. Do not immerse them in water — they soak up water like a sponge.

Store fresh mushrooms in the refrigerator for up to 1 week in a paper bag rather than in plastic, where they are too moist and become slimy.

Nutritional value
Per serving

Calories	434
Protein	27 g
Fat	6 g
Carbohydrate	64 g
Dietary Fiber (a very high source)	7 g
Calcium (a source)	138 mg

Percent of calories from

Protein	25%
Fat	13%
Carbohydrate	58%

- Preheat oven to 425°F (220°C)
- 10-inch (25 cm) pie plate, sprayed with nonstick baking spray

Potato Shell

6	medium potatoes, peeled (about 2¼ lbs/1.125 kg)	6
1 cup	lactose-free milk or fortified soy milk	250 mL
½ tsp	salt	2 mL
Pinch	ground nutmeg	Pinch
Pinch	freshly ground black pepper	Pinch

Fish Filling

1½ cups	water	375 mL
½ cup	dry white wine	125 mL
1	bay leaf	1
1	carrot, coarsely chopped	1
1	stalk celery, coarsely chopped	1
1	onion, stuck with 4 whole cloves	1
1 lb	sole or haddock, fresh or frozen	500 g
1 tbsp	vegetable oil	15 mL
4 oz	mushrooms, sliced	125 g
1 cup	sliced leek	250 mL
2 tbsp	all-purpose flour	25 mL
	Salt and freshly ground black pepper	

1. *Prepare the Potato Shell:* In a large saucepan, cover potatoes with cold water and bring to a boil over high heat; reduce heat to medium and simmer for 20 to 25 minutes, or until tender. Drain and mash with a fork or potato masher. Beat in milk, salt, nutmeg and pepper until fluffy. Spread over bottom and sides of prepared pie plate, making decorative swirls.

2. *Prepare the Fish Filling:* Meanwhile, in another large saucepan, bring water, wine, bay leaf, carrot, celery and onion stuck with cloves to a boil over high heat. Reduce heat to medium and simmer for about 15 minutes to allow flavors to blend.

3. Add fish, cutting into large chunks if necessary to fit, and bring to a boil over medium heat. Reduce heat to low and simmer until fish flakes easily when tested with a fork, 5 to 10 minutes, depending on whether fish was fresh or frozen. Drain and reserve stock and fish. Discard vegetables and bay leaf.

4. In the same saucepan, heat oil over medium heat. Cook mushrooms and leeks until tender, about 5 minutes. Sprinkle with flour and stir until smooth. Remove from heat. Gradually whisk in reserved fish stock. Return to heat. Cook, stirring, until thickened, about 2 minutes. Stir in reserved fish and salt and pepper to taste.

5. Spoon filling into potato shell. Bake in preheated oven for 20 to 25 minutes, or until golden brown around edges. Cut into wedges to serve.

Variation

Coquilles St. Jacques: Substitute fresh sea scallops for the fish. Leave scallops whole, and reduce cooking time in Step 3 to 3 minutes, or just until scallops are opaque.

TIPS

For a richer flavor, substitute portobello mushrooms for button mushrooms.

Because leeks are grown mounded in sand, they often have grit or sand between the layers. To clean leeks, slice them lengthwise almost to the root and let tap water run through the various layers, removing any sand or grit.

Easy Salmon Pie

With prepared pie shells and canned salmon, this party dish is a snap to make. It is delicious served with Dill Mustard Sauce (see recipe, page 246).

MAKES 6 SERVINGS

TIPS

This is a simple takeoff on the classic Russian dish kulebiaka, made with a rich sour cream and butter pastry. Serve this elegant pie with Green Sauce (see page 245) and a salad of calcium greens.

Dill is a wonderful complement to salmon.

One lemon will yield about ¼ cup (50 mL) of juice, especially if you run the lemon under hot water or warm it in the microwave for about 10 seconds.

Nutritional value
Per serving

Calories	451
Protein	17 g
Fat	27 g
Carbohydrate	34 g
Dietary Fiber	1 g
Calcium (a high source)	196 mg

Percent of calories from

Protein	15%
Fat	55%
Carbohydrate	30%

● Preheat oven to 425°F (220°C)
● 9-inch (23 cm) pie plate

1 ½ cups	water	375 mL
¾ cup	mixed white and wild rice	175 mL
1	bay leaf	1
2 tbsp	vegetable oil	25 mL
1	onion, chopped	1
2	cans (each 7.5 oz/213 g) sockeye salmon	2
2	hard-cooked eggs, peeled and chopped	2
¼ cup	chopped fresh dill	50 mL
¼ cup	chopped fresh parsley	50 mL
¼ cup	freshly squeezed lemon juice	50 mL
½ tsp	salt	2 mL
¼ tsp	freshly ground black pepper	1 mL
2	unbaked 9-inch (23 cm) pie shells	2
1	egg, beaten with 1 tbsp (15 mL) water	1

1. In a medium saucepan, bring water to a boil over high heat. Cook rice and bay leaf until water is absorbed and rice is tender, about 25 minutes. Discard bay leaf.

2. In a small skillet, heat oil over medium-high heat. Cook onion, covered, until softened, about 5 minutes.

3. Meanwhile, drain salmon, discarding skin and mashing bones.

4. In a large bowl, combine rice, onion, salmon, eggs, dill, parsley, lemon juice, salt and pepper.

5. Gently press 1 pie shell into pie plate. Spoon in salmon mixture and top with the other pie shell. Crimp edges together with dampened fingers and make decorative air vents in the top. Brush with egg wash.

6. Bake in preheated oven for 10 to 15 minutes, or until pastry is starting to brown. Reduce temperature to 350°F (180°C) and cook until pastry is golden brown, about 30 minutes. Let cool for at least 15 minutes before serving. Serve hot or at room temperature.

TIP

If a full bunch of dill, parsley or any other fresh herb is more than you need for a recipe, wash, dry and chop whatever is left over, wrap it in plastic wrap, label it and freeze it for up to 1 year. It's the ultimate convenience for future recipes.

MAKE AHEAD

Cover and store in the refrigerator for up to 1 day.

Grilled Salmon

Preparing salmon for oven grilling or barbecuing takes minutes, and this dish doesn't require a buttery basting during cooking. A mere squeeze of lemon is all that is required to make this salmon perfect.

MAKES 1 SERVING

- Preheat oven to 450°F (230°C) (or preheat barbecue to medium-high)
- Baking pan, sprayed with nonstick baking spray (if using barbecue, spray a piece of foil)

4 oz	salmon fillet	125 g
1 tbsp	white wine	15 mL
2 tsp	chopped fresh tarragon or dill	10 mL
1 1/2 tsp	extra-virgin olive oil	7 mL
	Freshly ground black pepper	

1. Arrange salmon fillet skin side down in prepared baking pan. Sprinkle with wine, dill, olive oil and pepper.

2. Bake in preheated oven (or on grill) for 10 to 15 minutes, depending on thickness of fillet, until fish is opaque and flakes easily when tested with a fork.

Nutritional value
Per serving

Calories	176
Protein	16 g
Fat	11 g
Carbohydrate	1 g
Dietary Fiber	0 g
Calcium	22 mg

Percent of calories from

Protein	38%
Fat	55%
Carbohydrate	1%

Salmon Mousse

My adaptation of my mother's delicious recipe is lactose-free, but screams of cream! Serve it with Cucumber Almond Salad (see recipe, page 96) and bread, and garnish with sliced cucumber and lemon.

MAKES 4 CUPS (1 L) OR 6 SERVINGS

MAKE AHEAD

Store in the refrigerator for up to 1 day.

- 4-cup (1 L) mold or small loaf pan, lined with plastic wrap

1	package (10.25 oz/290 g) silken soft tofu	1
2	cans (each 7.5 oz/213 g) salmon	2
4 1/2 tsp	gelatin (about 1 1/2 envelopes)	22 mL
3 tbsp	freshly squeezed lemon juice	45 mL
1/2 cup	boiling water	125 mL
1/2 cup	light salad dressing	125 mL
1/4 cup	chopped fresh dill	50 mL
1/4 cup	chopped green onion	50 mL
1/4 tsp	freshly ground black pepper	1 mL

1. Using a sieve, drain tofu. Drain salmon, discarding skin and reserving bones.

2. In a small bowl, sprinkle gelatin over lemon juice. Let stand until lemon juice has been absorbed, about 5 minutes. Stir in boiling water until gelatin is dissolved.

3. In a food processor, combine drained tofu, salmon and bones, salad dressing, dill, onion and pepper; purée until smooth. With motor running, pour dissolved gelatin through feed tube and purée until combined.

4. Spoon salmon mixture into prepared pan; cover and refrigerate for about 2 hours, until firm. To unmold, place serving platter over mold; invert mold and, using plastic wrap as lever, gently ease mousse onto platter. Remove plastic wrap. Slice into 1/2-inch (1 cm) pieces.

Nutritional value
Per serving (2/3 cup/150 mL)

Calories	212
Protein	16 g
Fat	14 g
Carbohydrate	5 g
Dietary Fiber	0 g
Calcium (a high source)	183 mg

Percent of calories from

Protein	31%
Fat	60%
Carbohydrate	9%

Salmon Loaf

You can serve salmon loaf hot or cold. Try slicing chilled salmon loaf and serving it on pumpernickel as an appetizer.

TIPS

Canned salmon with the bones is an excellent source of calcium and vitamin D, both required for good bone health.

For perfect, fluffy bread crumbs, use a blender or food processor and tear bread slices into pieces before adding them to the machine.

Nutritional value
Per serving

Calories	277
Protein	17 g
Fat	14 g
Carbohydrate	19 g
Dietary Fiber	1 g
Calcium	246 mg
(a high source)	

Percent of calories from

Protein	25%
Fat	46%
Carbohydrate	28%

- Preheat oven to 350°F (180°C)
- 8½- x 4½-inch (1.5 L) loaf pan, lined with parchment paper

2	cans (each 7.5 oz/213 g) sockeye salmon	2
2	eggs	2
1 cup	fresh bread crumbs (about 2 slices)	250 mL
½ cup	light whipped salad dressing	125 mL
½ cup	lactose-free milk or fortified soy milk	125 mL
¼ cup	grated onion	50 mL
¼ cup	chopped fresh parsley	50 mL
2 tbsp	chopped fresh dill	25 mL
2 tbsp	freshly squeezed lemon juice	25 mL
½ tsp	salt	2 mL
¼ tsp	freshly ground black pepper	1 mL

1. Drain salmon, discarding skin and mashing bones.

2. In a medium bowl, thoroughly mix salmon and bones, eggs, bread crumbs, salad dressing, milk, onion, parsley, dill, lemon juice, salt and pepper. Spoon into prepared pan.

3. Bake in preheated oven for about 1 hour, or until puffed, golden and firm to touch. Let cool in pan on a wire rack, then gently remove salmon loaf from pan, using parchment paper as handles. Let stand for 10 to 15 minutes before slicing, or serve chilled.

Burgers with the Works

A barbecued hamburger with all the fixings is oh-so-delicious! The binding in commercial patties often contains lactose, but this recipe is lactose-free and produces a succulent burger in minutes.

MAKES 4 SERVINGS

TIP

It is no longer safe to serve rare beef burgers. They should be cooked until no longer pink inside; check doneness with the point of a sharp knife or use a meat thermometer.

Nutritional value	
Per serving	
Calories	413
Protein	29 g
Fat	19 g
Carbohydrate	29 g
Dietary Fiber (a source)	2 g
Calcium (a source)	89 mg
Percent of calories from	
Protein	29%
Fat	42%
Carbohydrate	29%

● *Preheat barbecue to medium-high*

1	slice French-style bread, torn into pieces	1
1	egg	1
1 lb	lean ground beef	500 g
2 tbsp	ketchup	25 mL
1 tsp	Worcestershire sauce	5 mL
½ tsp	salt	2 mL
¼ tsp	freshly ground black pepper	1 mL
4	hamburger buns	4
	Sliced tomatoes and onions	

1. In a blender or food processor, process bread pieces to fine crumbs.

2. In a medium bowl, combine bread crumbs, egg, ground beef, ketchup, Worcestershire sauce, salt and pepper. Mix well. Form into 4 patties, each 4 inches by ¾ inch (10 by 1.5 cm)

3. Place patties on preheated grill. Grill for about 12 minutes, turning twice, until patties reach an internal temperature of 170°F (75°C) and are no longer pink inside.

4. Meanwhile, toast buns on the barbecue.

5. Serve immediately on toasted buns, with tomato slices, onions and condiments of your choice.

Variation

If you prefer, substitute ground chicken or turkey for the beef. Grill to an internal temperature of 175°F (80°C).

Veal and Mushrooms

This hearty veal stew has a tantalizing flavor. Serve with Creamy Mashed Potatoes with Garlic (see recipe, page 170) and Nice 'n' Nutty Slaw (see recipe, page 102).

MAKES 8 SERVINGS

TIPS

Clean mushrooms with a damp cloth; do not immerse them in water, as they absorb water like a sponge.

Store fresh mushrooms in the refrigerator for up to 1 week in a paper bag rather than in plastic, where they are too moist and become slimy.

3 lbs	stewing veal	1.5 kg
2 cups	chicken stock (store-bought or see recipe, page 68)	500 mL
1	onion, studded with 6 whole cloves	1
1	carrot	1
1	stalk celery	1
1	bay leaf	1
½ tsp	dried thyme	2 mL
2 tbsp	vegetable oil	25 mL
1	large onion, sliced	1
8 oz	mushrooms, sliced	250 g
¼ cup	all-purpose flour	50 mL
2 tbsp	freshly squeezed lemon juice	25 mL
¼ cup	lactose-free milk	50 mL
½ tsp	salt	2 mL
¼ tsp	freshly ground black pepper	1 mL
¼ tsp	ground nutmeg	1 mL
	Chopped fresh parsley	

1. In a large saucepan, combine veal, stock plus enough water to cover meat, onion studded with cloves, carrot, celery, bay leaf and thyme. Bring to a boil over high heat; reduce heat to medium-low and simmer, uncovered, until veal is tender, about 1½ hours. Drain through a sieve, reserving veal and stock. Discard other solids.

Nutritional value
Per serving

Calories	495
Protein	55 g
Fat	24 g
Carbohydrate	13 g
Dietary Fiber (a source)	2 g
Calcium (a source)	73 mg

Percent of calories from

Protein	45%
Fat	44%
Carbohydrate	11%

2. In the same saucepan, heat oil over medium-high heat. Cook onion and mushrooms, covered, until softened, about 5 minutes. Sprinkle with flour and cook, stirring, for 3 to 4 minutes, or until well combined and flour is browned. Gradually whisk in reserved stock and lemon juice. Increase heat to high and cook, uncovered, stirring frequently, for 8 to 10 minutes, or until thickened.

3. Reduce heat to medium and add veal to sauce. Stir in milk, salt, pepper and nutmeg. Cook until heated through, about 5 minutes. Taste and adjust seasoning as desired with more salt and pepper. Serve garnished with parsley.

Variation

Substitute boneless pork shoulder blade for the veal.

TIP

One half lemon will yield about 2 tbsp (25 mL) of juice, especially if you run the lemon under hot water or warm it in the microwave for about 10 seconds.

MAKE AHEAD

Spoon into an airtight container and store in the refrigerator for up to 2 days or in the freezer for up to 3 months.

Beef Stroganoff

This classic Russian dish, usually rich with sour cream, takes on a new face in this lactose-free recipe.

MAKES 4 SERVINGS

TIPS

Leftover tomato paste can be frozen in measured amounts in an ice cube tray, then packed in freezer bags, ready to add to recipes. Store in the freezer for up to 3 months.

Traditionally, sour cream is added to stroganoff. In this version, the natural sweetness of lactose-free milk works well as a substitution.

1 lb	sirloin steak, cut crosswise into 1/4-inch (0.5 cm) slices	500 g
2 tbsp	all-purpose flour	25 mL
2 tbsp	vegetable oil	25 mL
1	large onion, chopped	1
1	clove garlic, minced	1
8 oz	mushrooms, sliced	250 g
1 cup	beef stock	250 mL
2 tbsp	tomato paste	25 mL
2 tbsp	dry sherry (optional)	25 mL
1 tsp	Worcestershire sauce	5 mL
1/2 tsp	salt	2 mL
Pinch	freshly ground black pepper	Pinch
1/2 cup	lactose-free milk	125 mL
	Cooked rice or noodles	

1. In a medium bowl, toss beef slices in flour to coat.

2. In a large skillet, heat oil over medium-high heat. Stir-fry beef until browned, about 2 minutes. Remove beef to a plate, cover and set aside.

3. Add onion, garlic and mushrooms to skillet; cook, covered, until softened, about 5 minutes.

4. In a measuring cup, whisk together beef stock, tomato paste, sherry, Worcestershire sauce, salt and pepper. Stir into vegetable mixture and cook until heated through, about 1 minute.

5. Return meat to vegetable mixture. Stir in milk and cook, stirring, until heated through, about 1 minute. Taste and adjust seasoning as desired with salt and pepper.

6. Serve over rice or noodles.

Nutritional value
Per serving

Calories	348
Protein	37 g
Fat	16 g
Carbohydrate	12 g
Dietary Fiber (a source)	2 g
Calcium (a source)	81 mg

Percent of calories from

Protein	43%
Fat	43%
Carbohydrate	14%

Side Dishes

Who doesn't love that wonderful comfort food, mashed potatoes, or, for that matter, scalloped potatoes? This chapter provides recipes for these popular creamy vegetable dishes. In addition, it includes vegetable dishes containing available calcium — that is, calcium that can be absorbed by our bodies. There are a number of vegetables with this mineral, but only some of them have available calcium (see chart, page 22).

Quick Sauté of Collard Greens 160

Stir-fry of Greens 161

Braised Kale 162

Artichokes with Spicy
   Lemon Sauce 163

Broccoli Soufflé 164

Carrots with Maple Syrup 166

Loaf Pan Carrot Stuffing 167

Carrot Squash Crumble 168

Scalloped Potatoes 169

Creamy Mashed Potatoes
   with Garlic 170

Mashed Potato Casserole 171

Salmon-Stuffed Baked Potatoes 172

Risotto 173

New-Fashioned Bean Pot 174

Quick Sauté of Collard Greens

Collards are among the oldest of all relations to the cabbage and are a vegetable source of available calcium. They have a wonderful tangy taste that complements ham, pork and stew recipes. The large, dark green, paddle-shaped leaves need to have their tough stem removed before being boiled in water. Afterwards, they may be sautéed, as in this recipe, or combined with a béchamel sauce as a side dish.

MAKES 4 SERVINGS

1	bunch (12 oz/375 g) collard greens	1
1 tbsp	extra-virgin olive oil	15 mL
1	clove garlic, crushed	1

1. Remove the tough central collard stem. Boil leaves, uncovered, in large pot of water for about 15 minutes. Drain well and chop coarsely.

2. In a medium saucepan, heat oil over medium heat. Stir-fry collards and garlic for about 2 minutes to heat through. Serve at once.

Nutritional value
Per serving

(nutrient analysis shown for turnip greens, which are similar)

Calories	48
Protein	1 g
Fat	4 g
Carbohydrate	4 g
Dietary Fiber (a source)	3 g
Calcium (a source)	118 mg

Percent of calories from

Protein	8%
Fat	62%
Carbohydrate	30%

Stir-fry of Greens

Ready in minutes, this calcium-containing stir-fry is a delectable side dish or a quick vegetarian main course with the addition of crumbled tofu. Serve over basmati rice.

MAKES 4 SERVINGS

1	bunch (12 oz/375 g) bok choy	1
1	stalk broccoli ($1/3$ bunch)	1
1	stalk celery	1
$1/2$	green bell pepper, sliced	$1/2$
4 oz	mushrooms, sliced	125 g
2 tbsp	vegetable oil	25 mL
1	clove garlic, crushed	1
$1/2$ cup	water	125 mL
$1/4$ cup	soy sauce	50 mL
1 tsp	sesame oil	5 mL
2 tbsp	sesame seeds	25 mL

1. Slice bok choy into $1/2$-inch (1 cm) pieces. Cut broccoli into florets and slice the tender part of stem. Slice celery on the diagonal. Combine with green pepper and mushrooms and set aside.

2. In a wok or large saucepan, heat vegetable oil over medium-high heat. Stir-fry garlic for about 30 seconds. Add vegetables, stirring to coat. Add water and cook until tender-crisp, about 5 minutes. Stir in soy sauce, and sesame oil. Serve immediately with a sprinkle of sesame seeds.

Nutritional value
Per serving

Calories	143
Protein	5 g
Fat	10 g
Carbohydrate	10 g
Dietary Fiber (a high source)	4 g
Calcium (a source)	154 mg

Percent of calories from

Protein	13%
Fat	62%
Carbohydrate	25%

Braised Kale

Calcium-rich kale, a member of the cabbage family, has a piquant flavor and coarse texture that lends itself to this simple but tasty recipe — a wonderful accompaniment to roast pork. Although the bunches in the supermarket look huge, kale cooks down similar to spinach.

MAKES 4 SERVINGS

TIP

If you haven't tried kale yet, it's time to experiment with this calcium vegetable. Like spinach, kale contains calcium — a real plus for those on the lookout for alternative calcium sources. Unlike spinach, kale contains no oxalic acid, so nothing interferes with your ability to absorb the calcium. (See Bioavailability and Sources of Calcium, page 16.)

1	bunch kale, washed and tough stems removed	1
2 tbsp	extra-virgin olive oil	25 mL
1	clove garlic, crushed	1
	Salt and freshly ground black pepper	

1. In a large saucepan, bring about ½ inch (1 cm) water to a boil over high heat. Add kale and return to a boil; reduce heat to medium, cover and simmer for 3 to 4 minutes, or until limp. Drain well and chop coarsely.

2. In the same saucepan, heat oil over medium heat. Cook garlic until softened, about 1 minute. Add kale; cook, stirring, for 1 minute, until heated through. Season to taste with salt and pepper. Serve immediately.

Nutritional value
Per serving

Calories	101
Protein	4 g
Fat	8 g
Carbohydrate	8 g
Dietary Fiber (a high source)	4 g
Calcium (a source)	109 mg

Percent of calories from

Protein	12%
Fat	60%
Carbohydrate	28%

Artichokes with Spicy Lemon Sauce

I make this favorite appetizer all the time with a spicy lemon-butter mixture as a dipping sauce. However, for this cookbook, I came up with a lactose-free version using olive oil to replace the rich taste of butter — with great success! All preparation can be done ahead, then just a few last-minute touches are necessary. Try to find artichokes of a similar size.

MAKES 4 SERVINGS

TIPS

To eat these delectable morsels, pull off leaves one at a time; dip into sauce and drag the leaf through your teeth to remove the tender, delicate "meat" of the artichoke.

This sauce is wonderful with other vegetables too. Try it over broccoli or braised kale, collard, napa cabbage or bok choy.

Nutritional value Per serving	
Calories	170
Protein	5 g
Fat	12 g
Carbohydrate	16 g
Dietary Fiber (a high source)	4 g
Calcium (a source)	68 mg
Percent of calories from	
Protein	10%
Fat	57%
Carbohydrate	33%

4	medium artichokes	4

Spicy Lemon Sauce

2	cloves garlic, crushed	2
1/3 cup	freshly squeezed lemon juice	75 mL
1/4 cup	extra-virgin olive oil	50 mL
1 tsp	dried tarragon	5 mL
1 tsp	salt	5 mL
1 tsp	Worcestershire sauce	5 mL
1/4 tsp	freshly ground black pepper	1 mL
Pinch	cayenne pepper	Pinch

1. Using a sharp knife, cut 1/2 inch (1 cm) off the stem ends of the artichokes and the tips of leaves.

2. In a steamer over simmering water, steam artichokes for 35 to 40 minutes, or until very tender.

3. *Prepare the Spicy Lemon Sauce:* In a small saucepan, bring garlic, lemon juice, oil, tarragon, salt, Worcestershire sauce, pepper and cayenne to a boil over high heat; reduce heat to medium-low and simmer, uncovered, for 1 minute.

4. To serve, arrange artichokes in individual serving bowls. Spoon about 2 tbsp (25 mL) hot sauce over each serving of artichokes. Serve at once.

Broccoli Soufflé

Soufflés are easy to make, they look beautiful, and they taste divine. All in all, they are sure to impress! This version allows the lactose intolerant to enjoy them too.

MAKES 4 SERVINGS

TIP

If you prefer, buy whole nutmeg and grate it with a rasp (available at cookware stores). The taste of freshly grated nutmeg is far superior to that of packaged ground nutmeg. The rasp will also work well to grate the Parmesan cheese, not to mention the zest of citrus fruits.

Nutritional value	
Per serving	
Calories	414
Protein	27 g
Fat	24 g
Carbohydrate	27 g
Dietary Fiber (a very high source)	7 g
Calcium (a very high source)	432 mg
Percent of calories from	
Protein	25%
Fat	50%
Carbohydrate	25%

- Preheat oven to 400°F (200°C).
- 10-cup (2.5 L) soufflé dish or casserole dish, sprayed with nonstick cooking spray.

6 cups	broccoli florets and sliced peeled stems (1 bunch)	1.5 L
2 tbsp	vegetable oil	25 mL
2	cloves garlic, minced	2
1/4 cup	all-purpose flour	50 mL
1 cup	lactose-free milk or fortified soy milk	250 mL
1/4 cup	chopped fresh dill	50 mL
1/4 tsp	freshly ground black pepper	1 mL
Pinch	ground nutmeg	Pinch
3/4 cup	crumbled feta cheese (about 4 oz/125 g) (optional, if tolerated)	175 mL
6	egg yolks	6
7	egg whites	7
Pinch	salt	Pinch
1 tbsp	freshly grated Parmesan cheese (optional, if tolerated)	15 mL

1. In a large pot of boiling water, cook broccoli until tender-crisp, about 3 minutes. Rinse under cold water and drain.

2. In a large saucepan, heat oil over medium heat. Cook garlic, stirring, for 30 seconds. Stir in flour; cook for 1 minute. Gradually whisk in milk, dill, pepper and nutmeg. (Sauce will be very thick.) Remove from heat.

3. Stir feta cheese (if using) into sauce. Beat egg yolks into sauce. Stir in drained broccoli.

4. In a large bowl, using an electric mixer, beat egg whites and salt on high speed until soft peaks form. Fold one-quarter of the egg whites into the broccoli-cheese sauce. Gently fold in the remaining egg whites. Pour into prepared pan and sprinkle with Parmesan cheese (if using).

5. Bake in preheated oven for 35 to 40 minutes, or until puffed and golden brown on top. Serve immediately.

Variations

Substitute 8 cups (2 L) chopped stemmed kale (about 1 bunch) for the broccoli. Cook until wilted, about 5 minutes. Drain, rinse under cold water and press out excess moisture.

Substitute old Cheddar cheese for the feta.

TIPS

Some lactose-intolerant people can handle small quantities of feta and Parmesan without a problem. Whether to include cheese must be considered on an individual basis.

Always check eggs before using. Discard any with cracked shells, as they may carry the salmonella bacteria.

Leftover egg yolks can be used in scrambled eggs, French toast and custards. Store in an airtight container in the refrigerator for up to 2 days.

Carrots with Maple Syrup

A variation on glazed carrots, this version without butter is the perfect companion to an Easter menu.

MAKES 4 SERVINGS

2 lbs	carrots, peeled	1 kg
1½ cups	water	375 mL
¼ cup	pure maple syrup	50 mL
	Salt and freshly ground black pepper to taste	

1. Using a sharp knife, cut carrots into julienne strips, 4 inches by ¼ inch (10 cm by 0.5 cm).

2. In a large saucepan or Dutch oven, bring water to a boil over high heat. Add carrots and return to a boil; reduce heat to medium, cover and simmer for 3 to 4 minutes, or until tender-crisp. Drain.

3. Pour in maple syrup, stirring gently to combine. Return to a boil over high heat and boil, uncovered, for 2 to 3 minutes, until slightly thickened. Serve immediately.

Nutritional value
Per serving

Calories	139
Protein	2 g
Fat	0 g
Carbohydrate	34 g
Dietary Fiber (a very high source)	6 g
Calcium (a source)	79 mg

Percent of calories from

Protein	6%
Fat	3%
Carbohydrate	91%

Loaf Pan Carrot Stuffing

Baking a stuffing separately makes for a lighter, more easily digested dressing that has not absorbed the fat from the turkey. And, of course, it is easier to serve! This is a family favorite that's been modified using shortening and orange juice instead of my usual butter and milk. Almonds are added for calcium.

MAKES 1 LOAF (8 SERVINGS)

MAKE AHEAD

The dry ingredients for the stuffing can be assembled the night before, ready for the liquid ingredients to be added at the last minute.

Nutritional value
Per serving

Calories	343
Protein	9 g
Fat	17 g
Carbohydrate	42 g
Dietary Fiber (a high source)	4 g
Calcium (a source)	93 mg

Percent of calories from

Protein	10%
Fat	43%
Carbohydrate	47%

- Preheat oven to 350°F (180°C)
- 9- by 5-inch (2 L) loaf pan, greased

1 cup	all-purpose flour	250 mL
1 cup	fresh bread crumbs	250 mL
1	carrot, coarsely grated	1
½ cup	toasted chopped unblanched almonds (see tip, page 168)	125 mL
1 tsp	baking powder	5 mL
½ tsp	salt	2 mL
½ tsp	ground ginger	2 mL
½ tsp	ground nutmeg	2 mL
¼ cup	vegetable oil	50 mL
¼ cup	packed brown sugar	50 mL
1	egg	1
⅓ cup	fortified orange juice	75 mL

1. In a large mixing bowl, stir together flour, bread crumbs, carrot, almonds, baking powder, salt, ginger and nutmeg.

2. In a small bowl, beat together oil and sugar until fluffy; beat in egg and orange juice. Stir into dry ingredients just until moistened. Spoon into prepared loaf pan and cover with foil.

3. Bake in preheated oven for 50 to 60 minutes, or until firm to the touch and a toothpick inserted in the center comes out clean.

Carrot Squash Crumble

This oh-so-good casserole is almost like dessert. The crunchy nutty topping is an interesting contrast to the smooth interior of this make-ahead dish. For added speed, use frozen chopped squash, which requires no preparation and takes only minutes of cooking.

MAKES 8 TO 10 SERVINGS

TIP

Toasting nuts intensifies their flavor. To toast almonds, bake in preheated 350°F (180°C) oven for 10 to 12 minutes, or until golden brown and fragrant.

MAKE AHEAD

Prepare through Step 3, cover and store in the refrigerator for up to 2 days.

Nutritional value
Per serving (1/8th of recipe)

Calories	243
Protein	6 g
Fat	7 g
Carbohydrate	43 g
Dietary Fiber (a very high source)	7 g
Calcium (a source)	136 mg

Percent of calories from

Protein	10%
Fat	25%
Carbohydrate	65%

● Preheat oven to 350°F (180°C)
● 13- by 9-inch (3 L) baking dish, greased

2 lbs	butternut squash, peeled and coarsely chopped	1 kg
2 lbs	carrots, peeled and coarsely chopped	1 kg
3/4 cup	fortified orange juice	175 mL
2 tbsp	packed brown sugar	25 mL
1 tsp	salt	5 mL
1 tsp	ground cinnamon	5 mL

Nutty Topping

1 1/4 cups	fresh bread crumbs	300 mL
1/2 cup	toasted chopped almonds (see tip, at left)	125 mL
2 tbsp	olive oil	25 mL
1/2 tsp	salt	2 mL

1. In a large pot of boiling water, cook carrots and fresh squash for 25 to 30 minutes, or until very tender. (If using frozen squash, add to carrots for last 15 minutes of cooking.) Drain thoroughly.

2. Using a food processor or potato masher, purée vegetables. Beat in orange juice, brown sugar, salt and cinnamon. Spoon into prepared baking dish.

3. *Prepare the Nutty Topping:* In a small bowl, combine bread crumbs, almonds, oil and salt; sprinkle over casserole.

4. Bake, uncovered, in preheated oven for 50 to 60 minutes, or until piping hot.

Scalloped Potatoes

You can never have too much scalloped potato, so allow 2 potatoes per person. If there are any leftovers, they are a welcome addition to dinner the next night. This foolproof method ensures lots of creamy sauce to coat the potatoes.

MAKES 8 SERVINGS

TIP

Yukon Gold potatoes and baking potatoes make the best scalloped potatoes.

Nutritional value
Per serving

Calories	425
Protein	13 g
Fat	10 g
Carbohydrate	72 g
Dietary Fiber (a very high source)	6 g
Calcium (a very high source)	278 mg

Percent of calories from

Protein	12%
Fat	21%
Carbohydrate	67%

- Preheat oven to 350°F (180°C)
- 13- by 9-inch (3 L) baking dish, greased

5 lbs	potatoes, peeled and halved	2.5 kg
1/4 cup	all-purpose flour	50 mL
2 tbsp	vegetable oil	25 mL
6 cups	lactose-free milk or fortified soy milk	1.5 L
1 tsp	salt	5 mL
1/4 tsp	freshly ground black pepper	1 mL
1/4 tsp	ground nutmeg	1 mL
1/2 cup	fine dry bread crumbs	125 mL
2 tbsp	extra-virgin olive oil	25 mL
2 tbsp	freshly grated Parmesan cheese (optional, if tolerated)	25 mL

1. In a large saucepan, cover potatoes with cold water and bring to a boil over high heat. Reduce heat to medium, cover and simmer for 12 to 15 minutes, until barely tender. Drain well and let cool; slice thickly.

2. In the same saucepan, stir together flour and oil until smooth; cook over medium heat until starting to pull away from bottom of pan. Remove from heat. Gradually whisk in milk until smooth. Return to medium heat and cook, whisking frequently, until thickened. Whisk in salt, pepper and nutmeg.

3. Spoon potatoes into prepared baking dish and pour sauce over top.

4. In a small bowl, stir together bread crumbs, oil and cheese (if using) until well mixed. Sprinkle evenly over potatoes.

5. Bake in preheated oven for 30 to 35 minutes, or until heated through.

Creamy Mashed Potatoes with Garlic

For potato lovers who cannot have lactose, here are the best mashed potatoes.

MAKE AHEAD

Spoon into an airtight container and store in the refrigerator for up to 3 days. Reheat, covered, in the microwave on high for 6 to 8 minutes or in a 350°F (180°C) oven for 30 minutes, until piping hot.

2½ lbs	potatoes, peeled and cut into 2-inch (5 cm) chunks	1.25 kg
1	clove garlic	1
¼ tsp	salt	1 mL
¾ cup to 1 cup	lactose-free milk, fortified soy milk or chicken stock	175 to 250 mL
2 tbsp	extra-virgin olive oil	25 mL
¼ tsp	freshly ground black pepper	1 mL
	Chopped fresh parsley	

1. In a large saucepan, combine potatoes, garlic, salt and enough cold water to just cover potatoes. Bring to a boil over high heat; reduce heat to medium-low, cover and cook for 20 to 25 minutes, or until potatoes are very tender. Drain well and return potatoes to saucepan. Place over low heat to dry out potatoes slightly, shaking saucepan occasionally to prevent them from sticking.

2. Mash potatoes and garlic roughly with a fork. Using an electric mixer, beat potatoes with milk, oil and pepper until smooth and very creamy. Taste and adjust seasoning as desired with salt and pepper.

3. Serve immediately, sprinkled with parsley.

Variation

Substitute sweet potatoes for the white potatoes.

Nutritional value
Per serving

Calories	230
Protein	6 g
Fat	5 g
Carbohydrate	41 g
Dietary Fiber (a high source)	4 g
Calcium (a source)	86 mg

Percent of calories from

Protein	10%
Fat	20%
Carbohydrate	70%

Mashed Potato Casserole

Humble mashed potatoes have become chic food these days with added sautéed garlic to give zing. And for many people, the simple mashed potato of their childhood is a must to accompany Christmas dinner. Feel free to halve this recipe for a smaller quantity. If you want enough for leftovers, beat in a little more milk the next day to keep them at their creamy best.

MAKES 8 TO 10 SERVINGS

TIP

Don't try to short-circuit this recipe by using the food processor to mash potatoes: you will have glue before you know it. Mash with a potato masher or an electric mixer.

MAKE AHEAD

Prepare through Step 2 and store in the refrigerator for up to 2 days.

Nutritional value
Per serving (¹/₈th of recipe)

Calories	300
Protein	8 g
Fat	7 g
Carbohydrate	64 g
Dietary Fiber (a very high source)	6 g
Calcium (a source)	91 mg

Percent of calories from

Protein	10%
Fat	6%
Carbohydrate	84%

● Preheat oven to 350°F (180°C)
● 13- by 9-inch (3 L) baking dish, greased

5 lbs	baking potatoes, peeled and quartered	2.5 kg
2 cups	2% lactose-free milk	500 mL
1 tsp	salt	5 mL
½ tsp	freshly ground black pepper	2 mL
½ tsp	ground nutmeg	2 mL

1. In a large saucepan, cover potatoes with cold water and bring to a boil over high heat. Reduce heat to medium, cover and simmer for 20 to 25 minutes, or until very tender. Drain well.

2. Using an electric mixer or a potato masher, mash potatoes until smooth. Beat in milk, salt, pepper and nutmeg. Spoon into prepared baking dish and cover with foil.

3. Bake in preheated oven for 45 to 60 minutes, or until piping hot.

Salmon-Stuffed Baked Potatoes

This recipe is a nutrient powerhouse. The canned salmon (with mashed bones) is an excellent source of calcium and vitamin D, essential for the lactose intolerant, who cannot get these nutrients from dairy foods. The potato is a good source of fiber, vitamins and carbohydrate. What's more, this dish can be ready in minutes if you use a microwave!

MAKES 2 SERVINGS

TIP

Salmon bones contain calcium. Be sure to mash them well and include them whenever you use canned salmon. Discard the skin — its dark color and slippery texture distract from the salmon filling.

Nutritional value
Per serving

Calories	559
Protein	22 g
Fat	27 g
Carbohydrate	57 g
Dietary Fiber (a high source)	5 g
Calcium (a very high source)	278 mg

Percent of calories from

Protein	16%
Fat	44%
Carbohydrate	41%

- Preheat oven to 425°F (220°C) (optional)
- Baking sheet

2	large baking potatoes	2
1 tbsp	vegetable oil	15 mL

Salmon Filling

1	can (7.5 oz/213 g) sockeye salmon	1
1	stalk celery, diced	1
1	green onion, chopped	1
¼ cup	light mayonnaise	50 mL
¼ cup	chopped fresh dill	50 mL
1 tsp	grated lemon zest	5 mL
2 tbsp	freshly squeezed lemon juice	25 mL
¼ tsp	freshly ground black pepper	1 mL

1. Scrub potatoes, prick skins with a fork and brush with vegetable oil. Place on baking sheet and bake in preheated oven for about 1 hour, or until tender when pierced with the tip of a knife. (Or place on a microwave-safe plate and microwave on High for 20 minutes. Let stand for 2 minutes.)

2. *Prepare the Salmon Filling:* Drain salmon, discarding skin and mashing bones. In a medium bowl, stir together salmon with bones, celery, green onion, mayonnaise, dill, lemon zest, lemon juice and pepper until well combined.

3. Just before serving, cut a deep cross in the top of each potato; squeeze lightly to open. Spoon equal quantities of salmon mixture into each potato and serve immediately.

Risotto

This Italian rice specialty is typically rich with butter and cheese. This version has been made lactose-friendly with homemade chicken stock, olive oil and a small amount of aged cheese.

TIPS

Use kale, napa cabbage or broccoli for the calcium greens.

You may get to the desired consistency before you've used all the chicken stock.

Although homemade chicken stock is the best, to save time, look for quality homestyle chicken stocks in supermarkets.

1/4 cup	olive oil	50 mL
1	onion, finely chopped	1
1	leek (white and light green parts only), sliced	1
1 cup	Arborio rice	250 mL
1	bay leaf	1
1/2 cup	dry white wine (optional)	125 mL
1 tsp	salt	5 mL
1/4 tsp	freshly ground black pepper	1 mL
1/4 tsp	saffron	1 mL
4 cups	Basic Chicken Stock (approx.) (see recipe, page 68)	1 L
1 cup	finely chopped blanched calcium greens (see tip, at left)	250 mL
1/2 cup	toasted unblanched almonds (see tip, page 168)	125 mL
1 tbsp	grated lemon zest	15 mL
1/2 cup	freshly grated Parmesan cheese (optional, if tolerated)	125 mL

1. In a heavy saucepan, heat oil over medium-high heat. Cook onion and leek, covered, until softened, about 2 minutes. Stir in rice and cook, stirring, for 2 minutes. Stir in bay leaf, wine (if using), salt, pepper and saffron. Gradually stir in chicken stock, 1/2 cup (125 mL) at a time, stirring until all the stock is absorbed before adding more. Risotto is done when mixture is creamy and rice is just tender but slightly firm in the center. (Total cooking time will be 15 to 20 minutes.)

2. Discard bay leaf and stir in calcium greens, almonds and lemon zest. Spoon into serving bowls and sprinkle with Parmesan cheese, if tolerated.

Nutritional value
Per serving

Calories	526
Protein	15 g
Fat	25 g
Carbohydrate	66 g
Dietary Fiber (a source)	3 g
Calcium (a source)	122 mg

Percent of calories from

Protein	11%
Fat	42%
Carbohydrate	48%

New-Fashioned Bean Pot

A can of baked beans is a nutrition-packed time-saver. Navy beans, also called pea beans, the basis for baked beans, are a source of calcium. This quick recipe jazzes up a can of baked beans to give them a homemade taste. Serve with rice, Tortilla Chips (see recipe, page 35) or toast.

MAKES 4 SERVINGS

1 tbsp	vegetable oil	15 mL
1	large onion, chopped	1
1	green bell pepper, coarsely chopped	1
2	cans (each 14 oz/398 mL) beans in tomato sauce	2
¼ cup	salsa	50 mL

1. In a medium saucepan, heat oil over medium-high heat. Cook onion and green pepper, covered, for 4 to 5 minutes, or until softened. Stir in beans and salsa. Cook, stirring, until heated through.

Nutritional value
Per serving

Calories	246
Protein	8 g
Fat	4 g
Carbohydrate	44 g
Dietary Fiber (a very high source)	11 g
Calcium (a source)	73 mg

Percent of calories from

Protein	13%
Fat	16%
Carbohydrate	71%

Breads

Yeast Breads

Commercially produced yeast breads may contain milk solids, especially if they are made from a rich dough. Some people with lactose intolerance will be able to cope with bread containing milk products, while others will have symptoms. Only you can judge your individual sensitivity. Be sure to check the ingredients listed on the package for milk, milk solids, cheese flavor, whey, curds and some nondairy margarine. Avoid breads containing these products if you are sensitive. Breads that are generally safe for lactose-intolerant people are Italian or French stick, whole wheat and rye.

When making your own breads, you must use a hard wheat flour such as all-purpose or whole wheat, because of its gluten content. Gluten is a protein that gives the bread strength and the ability to rise and stretch. The other essential ingredient is yeast. You can buy it fresh or packaged in dried form. Dry yeast is probably the easiest to work with and is best stored in the refrigerator until the best-before date. You can always tell if yeast is still active by adding the lukewarm water and sugar in the recipe. It will become foamy and will have a distinctive beery smell. If it doesn't do anything, start again with a new yeast. Yeast breads are probably the easiest baking you could ever do. There is no need to feel intimidated — the breads are practically foolproof!

Quick Breads

Breads and other baked goods often rely on milk and butter because they have unique qualities that provide flavor, browning and sweetness. Milk also reacts with the leavening agents to make baked products rise nicely and stay risen. Baking without milk proved quite a challenge!

I found that fruit purées, fruit juice, coffee, beer, lactose-reduced milk and soy milk gave moisture. As I tested, I discovered a bonus: not only do fruit purées and fruit provide liquid, but using them often makes the fat content less than that of the original recipe.

The results are so scrumptious, you will want to start baking all your own breads!

Basic Yeast Bread 177
    Braided Loaf. 178
    Pan Buns. 178
    Bow Knots. 178
    Hamburger Buns. 179
    Crescent-Shaped Rolls 179
Herbed Spiral Loaf. 180
Swedish Tea Ring 181
Easy Health Bread 182
Celebration Bread 184
Whole-Grain Seed and Nut Bread. . . 186
Beer Bread 187
Double Cornbread 188
Blueberry Cornbread 189
Caraway Currant Soda Bread. 190
Banana Citrus Loaf. 191

Glazed Lemon Loaf 192
Orange, Almond and Apricot
    Tea Bread 193
Tropical Coffee Cake. 194
Pear Ginger Cake. 195
Sesame Tea Biscuits. 196
Lemon Sesame Twists 197
Orange Almond Scone 198
Currant Scones 199
Cranberry Apple Muffins 200
Good Morning Bran Muffins 201
Double Pumpkin Muffins. 202
Banana Bran Muffins with
    Cinnamon Sugar Topping. 203
Carrot, Apple and Almond Muffins . . . 204

Basic Yeast Bread

This is an easy, versatile recipe using all white or a mixture of whole-grain all-purpose flours. It has the flavor and texture of the rich sweet-dough recipes, but has no milk or butter added. Because it freezes well for up to 6 months, try making several of the variations that follow to sample at different times. This dough makes the best hamburger buns!

MAKES 3 LOAVES OR ABOUT 4 DOZEN ROLLS

TIP

The rising procedure may be speeded up by placing the bowl in a pan of warm water. Cover bowl with plastic wrap to create a cozy environment. Conversely, the process may be slowed down by placing the bowl in a cool spot.

3 cups	lukewarm water, divided	750 mL
1 tsp	granulated sugar	5 mL
2	packages (each ¼ oz/7 g) active dry yeast (2 tbsp/25 mL)	2
½ cup	vegetable oil	125 mL
½ cup	granulated sugar	125 mL
1 tbsp	salt	15 mL
9 cups	all-purpose flour (approx.)	2.25 L

1. Rinse a large bowl with hot tap water; drain. Pour in 1 cup (250 mL) of the lukewarm water; sprinkle with the 1 tsp (5 mL) sugar and yeast. Let stand until foamy and smelling like beer, about 10 minutes.

2. Whisk in the remaining lukewarm water, oil, the ½ cup (125 mL) sugar and salt. Whisk in about half of the flour, 1 cup (250 mL) at a time. Using a wooden spoon or kneading with floured hands, mix in enough of the remaining flour to make a stiff dough.

3. Knead dough until it is smooth, satiny and elastic and bounces back after a finger is pressed into it, about 4 minutes.

4. Clean bowl and wipe with vegetable oil. Return dough to oiled bowl, turning to grease all over. Let rise in a warm place (such as a turned-off oven with the light on) until doubled in size, 1 to 1½ hours.

5. Punch dough down and shape into any of the following recipes.

Variation

Whole Wheat Bread: Use half whole wheat flour and half all-purpose white flour.

Nutritional value
Per serving (¹⁄₂₄th of loaf)

Calories	76
Protein	2 g
Fat	2 g
Carbohydrate	13 g
Dietary Fiber	1 g
Calcium	3 mg

Percent of calories from

Protein	9%
Fat	20%
Carbohydrate	71%

MAKE AHEAD

Place in a large heavy-duty plastic bag and store at room temperature for up to 2 days. Or place in a doubled plastic bag and store in the freezer for up to 6 months.

Braided Loaf

A braided loaf makes an excellent hostess gift.

1. Brush a baking sheet with vegetable oil or spray with nonstick baking spray.

2. Using one-third of the Basic Yeast Bread dough, roll out into a 15- by 6-inch (38 by 15 cm) rectangle. Using a knife, cut lengthwise into 3 equal strands. Braid and tuck ends under.

3. Using a fork, beat 1 egg with 1 tbsp (15 mL) water; brush over dough. Sprinkle generously with sesame seeds.

4. Place on prepared baking sheet. Let rise in a warm place until doubled in size, about 1 hour. Meanwhile, preheat oven to 400°F (200°C).

5. Bake for 20 to 25 minutes, or until loaf is golden brown and sounds hollow when tapped on bottom. Let cool on a wire rack.

Pan Buns

When split and spread with your favorite sandwich filling, pan buns make a tasty change from the usual lunchtime sandwich. If made smaller, they are perfect for dinner rolls.

1. Brush muffin pans with vegetable oil.

2. Using one-third of the Basic Yeast Bread dough, divide into 12 equal portions for lunchtime buns or 18 for dinner rolls. Roll each into ball. Dip into bowl of sesame seeds.

3. Place each ball, sesame seed side up, in muffin pan. Let rise in a warm place until doubled in size, about 1 hour. Meanwhile, preheat oven to 400°F (200°C).

4. Bake for 12 to 15 minutes, or until buns are golden brown and sound hollow when tapped on bottom. Let cool on a wire rack.

Bow Knots

1. Brush a baking sheet with vegetable oil or spray with nonstick baking spray.

2. Using one-third of the Basic Yeast Bread dough, divide into 12 equal portions. Shape each into a 6 inch (15 mL) long rope. Tie loosely into a knot and tuck ends under. Dip into a bowl of sesame seeds.

3. Place knots about 2 inches (10 cm) apart on prepared baking sheet. Let rise in a warm place until doubled in size, 45 to 60 minutes. Meanwhile, preheat oven to 400°F (200°C).

4. Bake for 12 to 15 minutes, or until bow knots are golden brown and sound hollow when tapped on bottom. Let cool on a wire rack.

MAKES 8 BUNS

Hamburger Buns

These moist, slightly sweet buns contribute to a superb hamburger experience.

1. Brush a baking sheet with vegetable oil or spray with nonstick baking spray.

2. Using one-third of the Basic Yeast Bread dough, divide into 8 equal portions. Shape each into a ball.

3. Using a fork, beat 1 egg with 1 tbsp (15 mL) water; brush over dough balls. Dip each ball into a bowl of sesame seeds.

4. Place buns about 1 inch (2.5 cm) apart on prepared baking sheet. Let rise in a warm place until doubled in size, about 1 hour. Meanwhile, preheat oven to 400°F (200°C).

5. Bake for 12 to 15 minutes, or until buns are golden brown and sound hollow when tapped on bottom. Let cool on a wire rack.

MAKES 8 CROISSANTS

Crescent-Shaped Rolls

1. Brush a baking sheet with vegetable oil or spray with nonstick baking spray.

2. Using one-third of the Basic Yeast Bread dough, and using a rolling pin, roll out into a circle about ¼ inch (5 mm) thick. Using a knife, cut into 8 wedges. Starting from the outside edge, roll dough into the center; curve ends inwards.

3. Using a fork, beat 1 egg with 1 tbsp (15 mL) water; brush over dough.

4. Place rolls about 1 inch (2.5 cm) apart on prepared baking sheet. Let rise in a warm place until doubled in size, about 1 hour. Meanwhile, preheat oven to 400°F (200°C).

5. Bake for 12 to 15 minutes, or until rolls are golden brown and sound hollow when tapped on bottom. Let cool on a wire rack.

Herbed Spiral Loaf

A fragrant loaf spiraled with fresh chopped herbs makes a pretty slice — and sight.

MAKE AHEAD

Wrap in plastic wrap and store at room temperature for up to 2 days, or wrap in plastic wrap, then foil, and store in the freezer for up to 6 months.

● 9- by 5-inch (2 L) loaf pan, brushed with vegetable oil or sprayed with nonstick baking spray

Herb Filling

2 tbsp	extra-virgin olive oil	25 mL
2	cloves garlic, minced	2
1 cup	chopped green onions (about 4)	250 mL
1 cup	chopped fresh parsley	250 mL
2 tbsp	dried basil	25 mL
2 tbsp	dried tarragon	25 mL
1 tbsp	freshly squeezed lemon juice	15 mL
⅓	Basic Yeast Bread dough (see recipe, page 177)	⅓
	Egg wash (see tip, page 185)	
	Sesame seeds	

1. *Prepare the Herb Filling:* In a skillet, heat oil over medium heat; cook garlic, onions, parsley, basil and tarragon, covered, until herbs are softened, about 3 minutes. Stir in lemon juice.

2. Using a rolling pin, roll out Basic Yeast Bread dough into a 15- by 10-inch (38 by 25 cm) rectangle. Spread with herbs to within 1 inch (2.5 cm) of border. Starting from short end, roll up jelly-roll style, tucking ends under. Brush with egg wash and sprinkle with sesame seeds.

3. Place in prepared pan. Let rise in a warm place until doubled in size, about 40 minutes hour. Meanwhile, preheat oven to 400°F (200°C).

4. Bake for 25 minutes, or until loaf is golden brown and sounds hollow when tapped on bottom. Let cool on a wire rack.

Nutritional value
Per serving (¹⁄₁₆th of loaf)

Calories	56
Protein	1 g
Fat	3 g
Carbohydrate	8 g
Dietary Fiber	1 g
Calcium	20 mg

Percent of calories from

Protein	8%
Fat	39%
Carbohydrate	53%

Swedish Tea Ring

This is always a hit for brunch or with a cup of coffee.

MAKES 1 COFFEE CAKE

TIP

Toasting nuts intensifies their flavor. To toast almonds, bake in preheated 350°F (180°C) oven for 10 to 12 minutes, or until golden brown and fragrant.

MAKE AHEAD

Wrap in plastic wrap and store at room temperature for up to 2 days, or wrap in plastic wrap, then foil, and store in the freezer for up to 6 months.

Nutritional value
Per serving (¹⁄₁₆th of cake)

Calories	181
Protein	3 g
Fat	3 g
Carbohydrate	35 g
Dietary Fiber	1 g
Calcium	21 mg

Percent of calories from

Protein	7%
Fat	16%
Carbohydrate	77%

● Baking sheet, brushed with vegetable oil or sprayed with nonstick baking spray

⅓	Basic Yeast Bread dough (see recipe, page 177)	⅓
	Egg wash (see tip, page 185)	
½ cup	packed brown sugar	125 mL
½ cup	toasted chopped almonds (see tip, at left)	125 mL
½ cup	raisins or washed currants	125 mL
1 tsp	ground cinnamon	5 mL
½ tsp	ground nutmeg	2 mL

Glaze

¾ cup	sifted confectioner's (icing) sugar	175 mL
2 tbsp	freshly squeezed lemon juice	25 mL

1. Using a rolling pin, roll out dough into a 15- by 10-inch (38 by 25 cm) rectangle. Using a pastry brush, paint dough with egg wash.

2. In a small bowl, stir together brown sugar, almonds, raisins, cinnamon and nutmeg; sprinkle evenly over rectangle to within 1 inch (2.5 cm) of border. Starting from short end, roll up jelly-roll style. Form into a circle.

3. Place on prepared baking sheet. Using scissors, slash dough at 2-inch (10 cm) intervals three-quarters of the way through ring. Alternately arrange one piece in and one piece out of the circle. Cover loosely with a tea towel. Let rise in a warm place until doubled in size, about 1 hour. Meanwhile, preheat oven to 400°F (200°C).

4. Bake for 25 to 30 minutes, or until golden brown and firm to the touch. Let cool on a wire rack.

5. *Prepare the glaze:* In a small bowl, whisk together icing sugar and lemon juice; drizzle over cooled ring.

Easy Health Bread

This super-simple loaf requires a minimum of kneading and, as a result, is a coarse-grained bread that's ideal for toast or sandwiches. Bake two, one to eat now and another to freeze for future use.

MAKES 2 LOAVES

TIP

For added calcium, use all sesame seeds instead of mixed seeds, replace half of the bran with ½ cup (125 mL) soy flour, and substitute fancy molasses for the honey. Sesame seeds, soy flour and molasses are all sources of calcium (see chart, page 22).

● *Two 9- by 5-inch (2 L) loaf pans, greased*

3 cups	lukewarm water	750 mL
2 tsp	granulated sugar	10 mL
2	packages (each ¼ oz/7 g) active dry yeast (2 tbsp/25 mL)	2
¼ cup	packed brown sugar	50 mL
¼ cup	fancy molasses or liquid honey	50 mL
¼ cup	vegetable oil	50 mL
1 tbsp	salt	15 mL
6 cups	whole wheat flour (approx.)	1.5 L
1 cup	natural bran	250 mL
½ cup	wheat germ	125 mL
½ cup	quick-cooking rolled oats	125 mL
½ cup	mixed seeds such as sesame, poppy or pumpkin seeds	125 mL

1. Rinse a large bowl with hot tap water; drain. Pour in lukewarm water; sprinkle with sugar and yeast. Let stand until foamy and smelling like beer, about 10 minutes.

2. Whisk in brown sugar, molasses, oil and salt. Whisk in 3 cups (750 mL) of the flour, bran, wheat germ, oats and seeds. Beat in enough of the remaining flour to make a heavy, slightly wet dough. Flour hands and knead for 1 to 2 minutes.

Nutritional value
Per serving (¹⁄₂₄th of loaf)

Calories	92
Protein	4 g
Fat	3 g
Carbohydrate	15 g
Dietary Fiber (a source)	3 g
Calcium	33 mg

Percent of calories from

Protein	14%
Fat	24%
Carbohydrate	62%

3. Clean bowl and wipe with vegetable oil. Return dough to oiled bowl, turning to grease all over. Cover with a tea towel or plastic wrap. Let rise in a warm place until doubled in size, about 1 hour.

4. Punch down dough and knead with floured hands for about 1 minute. Divide in half, shape into loaves and place in prepared pans. Cover loosely with tea towels; let rise in a warm place until doubled in size, about 45 minutes. Meanwhile, preheat oven to 375°F (190°C).

5. Bake for 45 to 55 minutes, or until loaf is a deep golden brown and sounds hollow when tapped on bottom. Let cool in pans on wire racks for about 20 minutes, then remove from pans to racks to cool completely.

MAKE AHEAD

Wrap in plastic wrap and store at room temperature for up to 2 days, or wrap in plastic wrap, then foil, and store in the freezer for up to 6 months.

Celebration Bread

Wonderfully rich without the usual butter and milk, this sticky dough produces a moist, tender bread. It can be shaped into hot cross buns for Easter, made into a German stollen or easily spooned into a Bundt pan for a special Christmas coffee cake.

MAKES 1 LOAF

TIPS

If a 14-cup (3.5 L) Bundt pan is not available, use a regular 12-cup (3 L) Bundt and an 8½- by 4½-inch (1.5 L) loaf pan instead.

To speed the rising action of dough, place the bowl in a pan of warm water. Cover with plastic wrap. Dough should be doubled in size in double-quick time!

Nutritional value
Per serving (¹/₂₄th of loaf)

Calories	193
Protein	3 g
Fat	6 g
Carbohydrate	32 g
Dietary Fiber (a source)	2 g
Calcium	23 mg

Percent of calories from

Protein	7%
Fat	28%
Carbohydrate	65%

● *Baking sheet or 14-cup (3.5 L) Bundt pan, greased*

1½ cups	lukewarm water, divided	375 mL
1	package (¼ oz/7 g) active dry yeast (1 tbsp/15 mL)	1
1 tsp	granulated sugar	5 mL
1	egg	1
½ cup	granulated sugar	125 mL
½ cup	vegetable oil	125 mL
1 cup	raisins	250 mL
½ cup	currants, washed, or candied peel	125 mL
½ cup	toasted chopped almonds (see tip, page 181)	125 mL
1 tbsp	grated lemon zest	15 mL
2 tsp	salt	10 mL
1½ tsp	ground cinnamon	7 mL
½ tsp	ground cloves	2 mL
½ tsp	ground cardamom	2 mL
½ tsp	ground nutmeg	2 mL
4 cups	all-purpose flour	1 L
	Egg wash (see tip, opposite)	

Glaze

¾ cup	sifted confectioner's (icing) sugar	175 mL
2 tbsp	freshly squeezed lemon juice	25 mL
	Slivered almonds (optional)	

1. Rinse a large bowl with hot tap water; drain. Pour in ½ cup (125 mL) of the lukewarm water; sprinkle with yeast and the 1 tsp (5 mL) sugar. Let stand until foamy and smelling like beer, about 10 minutes.

2. Gradually whisk in the remaining water, egg, the $\frac{1}{2}$ cup (125 mL) sugar, oil, raisins, currants, almonds, lemon zest, salt, cinnamon, cloves, cardamom and nutmeg. Whisk in flour, 1 cup (250 mL) at a time, using a wooden spoon when dough becomes heavy. Beat vigorously with spoon or knead with well-floured hands until well combined. Dough should be moist.

3. Clean bowl and wipe with vegetable oil. Return dough to oiled bowl, turning to grease all over. Cover loosely with a tea towel. Let stand in a warm place until doubled in size, $1\frac{1}{2}$ to 2 hours.

4. Punch dough down and knead with floured hands for 1 to 2 minutes. *For stollen,* form into an oval and fold over lengthwise. *For hot cross buns,* divide into 16 portions and shape into balls. Place on prepared baking sheet. *For Bundt,* place in prepared pan.

5. Let rise in a warm place until doubled in size, 1 to $1\frac{1}{2}$ hours. Meanwhile, preheat oven to 375°F (190°C). Brush dough with egg wash.

6. Bake for 30 to 35 minutes for stollen, 20 to 25 minutes for buns, 45 to 50 minutes for Bundt, or until bread is golden brown and sounds hollow when tapped on bottom. Let cool on a wire rack.

7. *Prepare the glaze:* In a small bowl, whisk together confectioner's sugar and lemon juice; drizzle over cooled bread. For hot cross buns, drizzle to make a cross. For stollen or Bundt, decorate with almonds, if desired.

TIP

Egg wash acts as a type of glue, usually to make seeds stick. Egg wash also gives a golden sheen to baked goods. To make egg wash, combine 1 beaten egg with 1 tbsp (15 mL) water. Use a pastry brush to paint egg wash onto the dough. Egg wash may be covered and stored in the refrigerator for up to 1 day.

MAKE AHEAD

Prepare through Step 7, wrap in plastic wrap, then in foil, and store in the freezer for up to 6 months.

Whole-Grain
Seed and Nut Bread

Make this bread in minutes and enjoy the results sliced and toasted with marmalade or as an accompaniment to soup and salad. It is excellent with Salmon Mousse (see recipe, page 153). When measuring the dry ingredients, be sure to spoon the flour into a dry measure and level with a knife to ensure correct amounts.

MAKES 1 LOAF

MAKE AHEAD

Cover and store in the refrigerator for up to 5 days, or wrap in plastic wrap, then foil, and store in the freezer for up to 3 months.

- Preheat oven to 350°F (180°C)
- 9- by 5-inch (2 L) loaf pan, lined with parchment paper

2 cups	all-purpose flour	500 mL
1 cup	whole wheat flour	250 mL
1 cup	quick-cooking rolled oats	250 mL
1 cup	natural bran	250 mL
½ cup	toasted chopped almonds or hazelnuts (see tip, page 181)	125 mL
¼ cup	sesame seeds	50 mL
2 tsp	baking powder	10 mL
1 tsp	baking soda	5 mL
1 tsp	salt	5 mL
1½ cups	fortified soy milk or lactose-reduced milk	375 mL
½ cup	liquid honey	125 mL

1. In a large bowl, stir together all-purpose flour, whole wheat flour, oats, bran, almonds, sesame seeds, baking powder, baking soda and salt. Using a fork, stir in milk and honey just until dry ingredients are moistened. Spoon into prepared pan.

2. Bake in preheated oven for 50 to 60 minutes, or until a tester inserted in the center comes out clean. Using parchment paper, lift bread out of pan onto a wire rack. Let cool before slicing.

Nutritional value
Per serving (½-inch/1 cm slice)

Calories	154
Protein	5 g
Fat	4 g
Carbohydrate	27 g
Dietary Fiber (a source)	3 g
Calcium	50 mg

Percent of calories from

Protein	13%
Fat	20%
Carbohydrate	67%

Beer Bread

Beer gives this bread a yeasty flavor and an unusual zing! It is an excellent companion to hearty soups such as Mushroom Chowder (see recipe, page 80).

MAKES 1 LOAF

MAKE AHEAD

Cover and store at room temperature for up to 2 days, or wrap in plastic wrap, then foil, and store in the freezer for up to 4 months.

- Preheat oven to 350°F (180°C)
- 9- by 5-inch (2 L) loaf pan, lined with waxed paper

2 cups	all-purpose flour	500 mL
1 cup	whole wheat flour	250 mL
¼ cup	loosely packed brown sugar	50 mL
1 tbsp	baking powder	15 mL
2 tsp	caraway or dill seeds	10 mL
1 tsp	salt	5 mL
1	bottle (12 oz/341 mL) beer	1
1 tbsp	additional caraway or dill seeds (optional)	15 mL

1. In a large bowl, stir together all-purpose flour, whole wheat flour, brown sugar, baking powder, caraway seeds and salt. Using a fork, stir in beer just until dry ingredients are moistened. Spoon into prepared pan and sprinkle with more seeds for garnish, if desired.

2. Bake in preheated oven for 55 to 60 minutes, or until a tester inserted in the center comes out clean. Let cool in pan on a wire rack before slicing.

Nutritional value
Per serving (½-Inch/1 cm slice)

Calories	92
Protein	3 g
Fat	0 g
Carbohydrate	19 g
Dietary Fiber	1 g
Calcium	18 mg

Percent of calories from

Protein	11 %
Fat	3%
Carbohydrate	80%

Double Cornbread

A moist bread with the rich sweetness of corn, this is ideal to pack for lunch or to serve with soup or salad.

TIPS

To cut cornbread, loosen edges with a knife, invert onto wire rack and remove waxed paper. Place serving plate on bread and invert. Cut into wedges.

Creamed corn replaces the milk in this recipe to give the necessary moisture.

MAKE AHEAD

Cover and store in the refrigerator for up to 2 days, or wrap in plastic wrap, then foil, and store in the freezer for up to 3 months.

Nutritional value
Per Serving (1/10th of cake)

Calories	129
Protein	2 g
Fat	7 g
Carbohydrate	16 g
Dietary Fiber	1 g
Calcium	16 mg

Percent of calories from

Protein	6%
Fat	45%
Carbohydrate	49%

● Preheat oven to 375°F (190°C)
● 9-inch (1.5 L) round cake pan, lined with waxed paper

1 cup	cake-and-pastry flour	250 mL
1 cup	cornmeal	250 mL
2 tsp	baking powder	10 mL
1 tsp	baking soda	5 mL
½ tsp	salt	2 mL
½ cup	shortening	125 mL
¼ cup	granulated sugar	50 mL
1	egg	1
1 cup	creamed corn	250 mL
½ cup	water	125 mL
	Sesame seeds	

1. In a medium bowl, stir together flour, cornmeal, baking powder, baking soda and salt.

2. In a separate bowl, using an electric mixer, beat together shortening and sugar until fluffy. Beat in egg, creamed corn and water until well combined. Using a fork, stir into dry ingredients just until moistened. Spoon into prepared pan and sprinkle with sesame seeds.

3. Bake in preheated oven for 30 to 35 minutes, or until firm to the touch and a tester inserted in the center comes out clean. Let cool in pan on a wire rack for about 15 minutes before removing paper (see tip, at left).

Variation

Double Cornbread Muffins: Spoon batter into 10 large muffin tins, lined with paper baking cups. Bake in preheated oven for 20 to 25 minutes.

Blueberry Cornbread

Make the most of fresh blueberries in this luscious breakfast or teatime treat. For more blueberry flavor, serve with Quick Blueberry Sauce (see variation, page 259).

(see variation, page 259)

MAKES 1 LOAF

TIP

For easy slicing, bake a day ahead of serving.

MAKE AHEAD

Cover and store in the refrigerator for up to 2 days, or wrap in plastic wrap, then foil, and store in the freezer for up to 2 months.

- Preheat oven to 350°F (180°C)
- 9- by 5-inch (2 L) loaf pan, lined with waxed paper

1 1/2 cups	all-purpose flour	375 mL
1 cup	cornmeal	250 mL
3/4 cup	granulated sugar	175 mL
2 tsp	grated lemon zest	10 mL
2 tsp	grated orange zest	10 mL
1 tsp	baking soda	5 mL
1/2 tsp	salt	2 mL
2	eggs	2
1/2 cup	fortified orange juice	125 mL
1/4 cup	vegetable oil	50 mL
1 1/2 cups	fresh blueberries	375 mL

1. In a large bowl, stir together flour, cornmeal, sugar, lemon zest, orange zest, baking soda and salt.

2. In a small bowl, whisk together eggs, orange juice and oil. Using a fork, stir into dry ingredients just until moistened. Fold in blueberries. Spoon into prepared pan.

3. Bake in preheated oven for 1 to 1 1/4 hours, or until firm to the touch and a tester inserted in the center comes out clean. Let cool in pan on a wire rack before slicing.

Nutritional value
Per serving (1/2-inch/1 cm slice)

Calories	139
Protein	3 g
Fat	3 g
Carbohydrate	25 g
Dietary Fiber	1 g
Calcium	7 mg

Percent of calories from

Protein	7%
Fat	22%
Carbohydrate	71%

Caraway Currant Soda Bread

Dazzle your friends with this quickly made bread. It's great served hot from the oven, cut into wedges or sliced and spread with Pear Butter (see recipe, page 253).

MAKES 1 LOAF

TIPS

This bread is at its best the day it is made.

Soaking currants cleans them and plumps them up, making them juicier in recipes.

MAKE AHEAD

Cover and store at room temperature for up to 2 days, or wrap in plastic wrap, then foil, and store in the freezer for up to 4 months.

Nutritional value
Per serving (½-inch/1 cm slice)

Calories	299
Protein	8 g
Fat	7 g
Carbohydrate	55 g
Dietary Fiber (a very high source)	7 g
Calcium	39 mg

Percent of calories from

Protein	10%
Fat	20%
Carbohydrate	70%

● *Preheat oven to 350°F (180°C)*
● *Baking sheet, greased*

¾ cup	currants	175 mL
3 cups	whole wheat flour	750 mL
1 cup	all-purpose flour	250 mL
2 tsp	baking powder	10 mL
1 tsp	baking soda	5 mL
1 tsp	salt	5 mL
1½ cups	water	375 mL
¼ cup	liquid honey	50 mL
¼ cup	vegetable oil	50 mL
2 tsp	caraway seeds	10 mL
	Granulated sugar	

1. In a small bowl, soak currants in warm water.

2. In a large bowl, stir together whole wheat flour, all-purpose flour, baking powder, baking soda and salt. Drain currants and add to bowl. Using a fork, stir in water, honey, oil and caraway seeds just until dry ingredients are moistened.

3. Knead with floured hands until smooth, about 1 minute. Shape into a 7-inch (18 cm) circle and place on prepared baking sheet. Cut a large X about ¼ inch (5 mm) deep on top; sprinkle with sugar.

4. Bake in preheated oven for about 1 hour, or until a tester inserted in the center comes out clean. Let cool on a wire rack for at least 10 minutes before slicing.

Banana Citrus Loaf

When you buy a bunch of bananas, there are always a few that become too ripe for eating. Save them for this recipe. Banana purée replaces milk in this recipe. Serve it sliced on its own or with Pear Butter (see recipe, page 253).

(see recipe, page 253)

MAKES 1 LOAF

TIP

If you don't feel like baking while bananas are at their peak of ripeness, freeze them for future use, skin and all. Simply peel and mash while still partially frozen.

MAKE AHEAD

Cover and store at room temperature for up to 4 days, or wrap in plastic wrap, then foil, and store in the freezer for up to 4 months.

Nutritional value
Per serving (½-inch/1 cm slice)

Calories	172
Protein	2 g
Fat	7 g
Carbohydrate	25 g
Dietary Fiber	1 g
Calcium	20 mg

Percent of calories from

Protein	5%
Fat	37%
Carbohydrate	58%

● Preheat oven to 350°F (180°C)
● 8½- by 4½-inch (1.5 L) loaf pan, lined with waxed paper

2 cups	cake-and-pastry flour	500 mL
2 tsp	baking powder	10 mL
1 tsp	baking soda	5 mL
½ tsp	salt	2 mL
½ tsp	ground nutmeg	2 mL
3	large ripe bananas, mashed	3
2	eggs	2
1 cup	lightly packed brown sugar	250 mL
½ cup	vegetable oil	125 mL
1 tbsp	grated orange zest	15 mL
1 tbsp	grated lemon zest	15 mL

1. In a large bowl, sift together flour, baking powder, baking soda, salt and nutmeg.

2. In a food processor or a medium bowl, combine bananas, eggs, brown sugar, oil, orange zest and lemon zest until smooth. Using a fork, stir into dry ingredients just until moistened. Spoon into prepared pan.

3. Bake in preheated oven for 55 to 60 minutes, or until firm to the touch and a tester inserted in the center comes out clean. Let cool in pan on a wire rack before slicing.

Glazed Lemon Loaf

A teatime favorite, this is excellent sliced and served with a cup of tea or fruit for dessert or brunch.

MAKES 1 LOAF

TIP

If you like, decorate the top of the loaf with slivers of orange and lemon peel before baking.

MAKE AHEAD

Cover and store in the refrigerator for up to 2 days, or wrap in plastic wrap, then foil, and store in the freezer for up to 4 months.

Nutritional value
Per serving (1/2-inch/1 cm slice)

Calories	131
Protein	2 g
Fat	5 g
Carbohydrate	20 g
Dietary Fiber	0 g
Calcium	17 mg

Percent of calories from

Protein	5%
Fat	34%
Carbohydrate	61%

- Preheat oven to 350°F (180°C)
- 8 1/2- by 4 1/2-inch (1.5 L) loaf pan, lined with waxed paper

1 1/2 cups	cake-and-pastry flour	375 mL
1 cup	granulated sugar, divided	250 mL
1 tsp	baking soda	5 mL
1/4 tsp	salt	1 mL
2	eggs	2
1/2 cup	lactose-reduced milk or fortified soy milk	125 mL
1/3 cup	vegetable oil	75 mL
1 tbsp	grated lemon zest	15 mL
1/4 cup	freshly squeezed lemon juice	50 mL

1. In a medium bowl, sift together flour, 3/4 cup (175 mL) of the granulated sugar, baking soda and salt.

2. In a small bowl, whisk together eggs, milk, oil and lemon zest. Using a fork, stir into dry ingredients just until moistened. Spoon into prepared pan.

3. Bake in preheated oven for 45 to 50 minutes, or until a tester inserted in the center comes out clean. Let cool in pan on a wire rack for about 15 minutes.

4. In a small bowl, whisk together the remaining sugar and lemon juice; pour over loaf while still warm in pan. Let cool completely before slicing.

Orange, Almond and Apricot Tea Bread

Apricots and almonds make a classic marriage of flavors. This is one of my favorite recipes, perfect with a cup of tea.

MAKES 1 LOAF

TIP

Sharp kitchen scissors make a fast job of cutting dried apricots.

MAKE AHEAD

Cover and store at room temperature for up to 3 days, or wrap in plastic wrap, then foil, and store in the freezer for up to 4 months.

Nutritional value
Per serving (½-inch/1 cm slice)

Calories	148
Protein	3 g
Fat	3 g
Carbohydrate	28 g
Dietary Fiber (a source)	2 g
Calcium	20 mg

Percent of calories from

Protein	8%
Fat	19%
Carbohydrate	74%

● Preheat oven to 350°F (180°C)
● 9- by 5-inch (2 L) loaf pan, lined with waxed paper

1 cup	dried apricots	250 mL
2 cups	all-purpose flour	500 mL
1 cup	granulated sugar	250 mL
½ cup	toasted chopped unblanched almonds (see tip, page 195)	125 mL
1 tsp	cream of tartar	5 mL
1 tsp	baking soda	5 mL
½ tsp	salt	2 mL
1	egg	1
¾ cup	fortified orange juice	175 mL
2 tbsp	vegetable oil	25 mL
1 tbsp	grated orange zest	15 mL
½ tsp	almond extract	2 mL

1. Pour boiling water over apricots; let stand for about 1 minute. Drain and chop.

2. In a large bowl, stir together flour, sugar, almonds, cream of tartar, baking soda and salt.

3. In a small bowl, whisk together egg, apricots, orange juice, oil, orange zest and almond extract. Using a fork, stir into dry ingredients just until moistened. Spoon into prepared pan.

4. Bake in preheated oven for 55 to 60 minutes, or until firm to the touch and a tester inserted in the center comes out clean. Let cool in pan on a wire rack before slicing.

Tropical Coffee Cake

This is an excellent recipe for using up the last overripe banana. Make it in winter when citrus fruits are at their peak and you need to be transported to a southern clime.

MAKES 1 CAKE

MAKE AHEAD

Cover and store at room temperature for up to 2 days, or wrap in plastic wrap, then foil, and store in the freezer for up to 4 months.

- Preheat oven to 350°F (180°C)
- 10-inch (3 L) Bundt pan, greased or sprayed with nonstick baking spray

1 cup	whole wheat flour	250 mL
1 cup	all-purpose flour	250 mL
¾ cup	granulated sugar	175 mL
1 tsp	baking soda	5 mL
1 tsp	baking powder	5 mL
½ tsp	salt	2 mL
2	eggs	2
1	ripe banana, mashed	1
1 cup	undrained crushed pineapple	250 mL
¼ cup	vegetable oil	50 mL
1 tbsp	grated orange zest	15 mL

1. In a large bowl, stir together whole wheat flour, all-purpose flour, sugar, baking soda, baking powder and salt.

2. In a small bowl, beat together eggs, banana, pineapple, oil and orange zest. Using a fork, stir into dry ingredients just until moistened. Spoon into prepared pan.

3. Bake in preheated oven for 50 to 60 minutes, or until firm to the touch and a tester inserted in the center comes out clean. Let cool in pan on a wire rack before slicing.

Nutritional value
Per serving (¹⁄₂₀th of cake)

Calories	113
Protein	2 g
Fat	3 g
Carbohydrate	20 g
Dietary Fiber	1 g
Calcium	10 mg

Percent of calories from

Protein	8%
Fat	23%
Carbohydrate	69%

Pear Ginger Cake

Be sure to slice the pears thinly for this recipe. You will find the batter stiff and heavy, but the pears give moisture during baking.

TIP

Toasting nuts intensifies their flavor. To toast almonds, bake in preheated 350°F (180°C) oven for 10 to 12 minutes, or until golden brown and fragrant.

MAKE AHEAD

Cover and store at room temperature for up to 2 days, or wrap in plastic wrap, then foil, and store in the freezer for up to 4 months.

Nutritional value
Per serving (¹⁄₂₀th of cake)

Calories	165
Protein	3 g
Fat	7 g
Carbohydrate	24 g
Dietary Fiber (a source)	2 g
Calcium	14 mg

Percent of calories from

Protein	6%
Fat	38%
Carbohydrate	56%

- Preheat oven to 350°F (180°C)
- 10-inch (3 L) Bundt pan, greased or sprayed with nonstick baking spray

1 cup	whole wheat flour	250 mL
1 cup	all-purpose flour	250 mL
1 cup	granulated sugar	250 mL
1 tsp	baking soda	5 mL
1 tsp	ground ginger	5 mL
½ tsp	ground nutmeg	2 mL
½ tsp	salt	2 mL
2 cups	thinly sliced peeled pears	500 mL
2	eggs	2
½ cup	vegetable oil	125 mL
¼ cup	toasted chopped almonds (see tip, at left)	50 mL
¼ cup	chopped crystallized ginger	50 mL
1 tbsp	grated lemon zest	15 mL
1 tbsp	freshly squeezed lemon juice	15 mL

1. In a large bowl, stir together whole wheat flour, all-purpose flour, sugar, baking soda, ground ginger, nutmeg, and salt. Add pears.

2. In a small bowl, whisk together eggs, oil, almonds, crystallized ginger and lemon zest and juice. Using a fork, stir into dry ingredients just until moistened. Spoon into prepared pan.

3. Bake in preheated oven for 60 to 70 minutes, or until a tester inserted in the center comes out clean. Let cool in pan on a wire rack for at least 15 minutes. Remove from pan and let cool completely on rack before slicing.

Sesame Tea Biscuits

After years of experimenting, I think this recipe makes the ultimate tender, flaky biscuits, the perfect companion to soups and salads.

MAKES 9 LARGE OR 12 MEDIUM BISCUITS

TIP

For tender biscuits, handle dough as little as possible. To keep dough from sticking to hands and cutter, lightly flour and wipe excess dough from hands and cutter between shaping.

MAKE AHEAD

Place in an airtight container and store in the refrigerator for up to 1 day or in the freezer for up to 3 months.

Nutritional value
Per serving (1 large biscuit)

Calories	231
Protein	4 g
Fat	13 g
Carbohydrate	24 g
Dietary Fiber (a source)	25 g
Calcium (a source)	59 mg

Percent of calories from

Protein	7%
Fat	51%
Carbohydrate	42%

- Preheat oven to 425°F (220°C)
- Baking sheet, greased or lined with parchment paper
- 2½-inch (6 cm) cookie cutter (optional)

2 cups	all-purpose flour	500 mL
2 tsp	cream of tartar	10 mL
2 tsp	granulated sugar	10 mL
1 tsp	baking soda	5 mL
½ tsp	salt	2 mL
½ cup	water	125 mL
½ cup	shortening, cubed	125 mL
½ cup	plain yogurt (if tolerated) or 1 cup (250 mL) fortified soy milk or lactose-reduced milk	125 mL
	Sesame seeds	

1. In a large bowl, stir together flour, cream of tartar, sugar, baking soda and salt. Using a pastry blender or 2 knives, cut in shortening until mixture resembles coarse crumbs. Using a fork, stir water and yogurt into dry ingredients just until moistened.

2. Turn out onto a lightly floured piece of waxed paper and pat into a circle about 1 inch (2.5 cm) thick. Using cookie cutter, cut dough into 9 biscuits; arrange on prepared baking sheet. (Or transfer whole circle to baking sheet and cut into wedges.) Brush lightly with water and sprinkle with sesame seeds.

3. Bake in preheated oven for about 15 minutes, or until golden brown on bottom. Serve immediately.

Variation

Savory Sesame Biscuits: For a zesty version, add ¼ cup (50 mL) chopped sun-dried tomatoes and 1 tsp (5 mL) dried basil to flour mixture.

Lemon Sesame Twists

These twists are a welcome addition to a bread basket for breakfast, lunch or dinner.

TIPS

Shortening does not need to be refrigerated and is easier to work with at room temperature.

Check egg cartons for date code to use before expiry date. Discard any eggs with cracks.

MAKE AHEAD

Place in an airtight container and store at room temperature for up to 1 day or in the freezer for up to 3 months.

Nutritional value
Per serving (1 biscuit)

Calories	203
Protein	5 g
Fat	10 g
Carbohydrate	23 g
Dietary Fiber	1 g
Calcium (a source)	65 mg

Percent of calories from

Protein	9%
Fat	45%
Carbohydrate	46%

● Preheat oven to 425°F (220°C)
● Baking sheet, greased

2½ cups	all-purpose flour	625 mL
1 tbsp	granulated sugar	15 mL
1 tbsp	grated lemon zest	15 mL
2 tsp	baking powder	10 mL
½ tsp	salt	2 mL
½ tsp	baking soda	2 mL
½ cup	shortening	125 mL
1	egg, beaten	1
1 cup	plain yogurt (if tolerated), fortified soy milk or lactose-reduced milk	250 mL
	Sesame seeds	

1. In a large bowl, stir together flour, sugar, lemon zest, baking powder, salt and baking soda. Using a pastry blender or 2 knives, cut in shortening until mixture resembles coarse crumbs.

2. In a small bowl, whisk together egg and yogurt. Reserving about 1 tbsp (15 mL) of the mixture, add the remainder to dry ingredients, stirring with fork just until moistened.

3. Divide into 12 equal pieces. Roll each piece into a rope and tie into a knot, tucking ends under. Place on prepared baking sheet. Brush with reserved egg mixture and sprinkle with sesame seeds.

4. Bake in preheated oven for 20 to 25 minutes, or until golden brown and firm to the touch. Serve hot or at room temperature.

Variation

Lemon Sesame Cake: After Step 2, spoon batter into a 9-inch (23 cm) round cake pan, lined with waxed paper. Continue with recipe, adding 5 minutes to the baking time.

Orange Almond Scone

A scone, traditionally made with cream and butter, is a rich cousin to the tea biscuit. However, this relative boasts orange juice and shortening to produce melt-in-your-mouth perfection.

MAKES 8 TO 12 WEDGES

MAKE AHEAD

Prepare through Step 2, cover with plastic wrap and store in the refrigerator for up to 12 hours. Remove from the refrigerator 30 minutes before baking.

Nutritional value
Per serving (⅛th of scone)

Calories	283
Protein	6 g
Fat	12 g
Carbohydrate	39 g
Dietary Fiber	1 g
Calcium	36 mg

Percent of calories from

Protein	8%
Fat	37%
Carbohydrate	55%

- Preheat oven to 400°F (200°C)
- 9-inch (23 cm) round cake pan, bottom lined with waxed paper

2 cups	all-purpose flour	500 mL
½ cup	granulated sugar	125 mL
1 tbsp	grated orange zest	15 mL
2 tsp	baking powder	10 mL
½ tsp	baking soda	2 mL
½ tsp	salt	2 mL
⅓ cup	shortening	75 mL
2	eggs	2
½ cup	fortified orange juice	125 mL
¼ cup	chopped almonds	50 mL

1. In a large bowl, stir together flour, all but 1 tbsp (15 mL) of the sugar, orange zest, baking powder, baking soda and salt. Using a pastry blender or 2 knives, cut in shortening until mixture resembles coarse crumbs.

2. In a small bowl, whisk together eggs and orange juice. Reserving 1 tbsp (15 mL) of the orange juice mixture, add the remainder to dry ingredients, stirring with fork just until moistened. Spoon into prepared pan and brush with reserved orange juice mixture. Sprinkle evenly with reserved sugar and almonds.

3. Bake in preheated oven for 25 to 30 minutes, or until golden brown and firm to touch. Let cool in pan on a wire rack for about 10 minutes. Run a knife around sides of pan to loosen and remove from pan. Cut into wedges and serve warm.

Currant Scones

The dessert version of tea biscuits, scones are usually made with butter, cream or sour cream. This lactose-free version is best served with Quick Strawberry Sauce (see recipe, page 259) or split and filled with sliced fresh berries as shortcake served with drained Yogurt Sauce (see recipe, page 256).

MAKES 12 TO 14 SMALL SCONES

TIP

For super easy biscuits, spoon dough into 10 greased muffin cups and bake for 15 to 20 minutes, or until firm to touch. No fuss, no muss!

MAKE AHEAD

Place in an airtight container and store in the refrigerator for up to 1 day or in the freezer for up to 3 months.

Nutritional value
Per serving (1 of 12 scones)

Calories	160
Protein	2 g
Fat	9 g
Carbohydrate	18 g
Dietary Fiber	1 g
Calcium	22 mg

Percent of calories from

Protein	5%
Fat	49%
Carbohydrate	46%

- Preheat oven to 425°F (220°C)
- Baking sheet, greased
- 1½-inch (4 cm) cookie cutter

2 cups	cake-and-pastry flour	500 mL
2 tbsp	granulated sugar	25 mL
2 tsp	cream of tartar	10 mL
1 tsp	baking soda	5 mL
½ tsp	salt	2 mL
½ cup	shortening, cubed	125 mL
½ cup	water	125 mL
½ cup	plain yogurt (if tolerated) or ⅔ cup (150 mL) lactose-reduced milk	125 mL
½ cup	currants, washed	125 mL
	Granulated sugar	

1. In a large bowl, stir together flour, sugar, cream of tartar, baking soda and salt. Using a pastry blender or 2 knives, cut in shortening until mixture resembles coarse crumbs. Using a fork, stir water, yogurt and currants into dry ingredients just until moistened.

2. Turn out onto a lightly floured sheet of waxed paper and pat into circle about 1 inch (2.5 cm) thick. Using cookie cutter, cut dough into 12 biscuits; arrange on prepared baking sheet. (Or transfer whole circle to baking sheet and cut into wedges.) Brush lightly with water and sprinkle with sugar.

3. Bake in preheated oven for 12 to 15 minutes, or until golden brown on bottom. Serve immediately.

Cranberry Apple Muffins

This not-too-sweet muffin is ideal to pack in lunches or to munch for breakfast.

MAKES 12 LARGE MUFFINS

TIP

Cardamom is a member of the ginger family and has a delightful flavor and fragrance. It is frequently used in Scandinavian baking and East Indian dishes.

MAKE AHEAD

Place in an airtight container and store at room temperature for up to 1 day or in the freezer for up to 4 months.

Nutritional value
Per serving (1 muffin)

Calories	247
Protein	3 g
Fat	10 g
Carbohydrate	36 g
Dietary Fiber	1 g
Calcium	12 mg

Percent of calories from

Protein	5%
Fat	37%
Carbohydrate	58%

- Preheat oven to 400°F (200°C)
- 12-cup muffin tin, greased or lined with paper baking cups

2 cups	all-purpose flour	500 mL
1 cup	granulated sugar	250 mL
1 tbsp	grated orange zest	15 mL
1 tsp	ground cinnamon	5 mL
1 tsp	baking soda	5 mL
1/2 tsp	salt	2 mL
1/4 tsp	ground nutmeg	1 mL
1/4 tsp	ground cardamom	1 mL
2	eggs	2
1 cup	unsweetened applesauce	250 mL
1 cup	fresh or frozen cranberries	250 mL
1/2 cup	vegetable oil	125 mL

1. In a large bowl, stir together flour, sugar, orange zest, cinnamon, baking soda, salt, nutmeg and cardamom.

2. In a medium bowl, whisk together eggs, applesauce, cranberries and oil. Using a fork, stir into dry ingredients just until moistened. Spoon into prepared muffin cups.

3. Bake in preheated oven for 15 to 20 minutes, or until tops spring back when lightly touched.

Good Morning Bran Muffins

Here's a hearty muffin to get the morning off to a good start.

MAKE AHEAD

Place in an airtight container and store at room temperature for up to 2 days or in the freezer for up to 4 months.

Nutritional value
Per serving (1 muffin)

Calories	272
Protein	5 g
Fat	6 g
Carbohydrate	55 g
Dietary Fiber (a high source)	4 g
Calcium (a source)	132 mg

Percent of calories from

Protein	6%
Fat	18%
Carbohydrate	75%

- Preheat oven to 375°F (190°C)
- 12-cup muffin tin, greased or lined with paper baking cups

1 cup	whole wheat flour	250 mL
1 cup	all-purpose flour	250 mL
1 cup	natural bran	250 mL
1 cup	packed brown sugar	250 mL
1 tsp	baking powder	5 mL
1 tsp	baking soda	5 mL
1 tsp	ground cinnamon	5 mL
1/2 tsp	salt	2 mL
1 cup	boiling coffee	250 mL
8 oz	dates, chopped (1 1/4 cups/300 mL)	250 g
1/2 cup	fancy molasses	125 mL
1/4 cup	vegetable oil	50 mL
1 tbsp	grated orange zest	15 mL
2	eggs, beaten	2

1. In a large bowl, stir together whole wheat flour, all-purpose flour, bran, brown sugar, baking powder, baking soda, cinnamon and salt.

2. In a medium bowl, pour boiling coffee over dates. Stir in molasses, oil and orange zest. Add to dry ingredients all at once. Add eggs and stir with a fork just until dry ingredients are moistened. Spoon into prepared muffin cups.

3. Bake in preheated oven for 20 to 25 minutes, or until tops spring back when lightly touched.

Double Pumpkin Muffins

Served with Pumpkin Butter (see recipe, page 252) or spread with honey, these muffins are wonderful packed in a lunch or as breakfast to go.

MAKES 12 LARGE MUFFINS

MAKE AHEAD

Place in an airtight container and store at room temperature for up to 2 days or in the freezer for up to 4 months.

Nutritional value
Per serving (1 muffin)

Calories	204
Protein	6 g
Fat	9 g
Carbohydrate	27 g
Dietary Fiber (a high source)	4 g
Calcium (a source)	59 mg

Percent of calories from

Protein	11%
Fat	38%
Carbohydrate	51%

● *Preheat oven to 375°F (190°C)*
● *12-cup muffin tin, greased or lined with paper baking cups*

1 cup	all-purpose flour	250 mL
1 cup	whole wheat flour	250 mL
1 tsp	baking soda	5 mL
1 tsp	baking powder	5 mL
1 tsp	ground cinnamon	5 mL
½ tsp	ground nutmeg	2 mL
½ tsp	ground cloves	2 mL
½ tsp	salt	2 mL
1	egg	1
1 cup	pumpkin purée (not pie filling)	250 mL
¾ cup	fortified soy milk or lactose-reduced milk	175 mL
½ cup	packed brown sugar	125 mL
½ cup	pumpkin seeds	125 mL
½ cup	currants, washed	125 mL
¼ cup	vegetable oil	50 mL
¼ cup	sesame seeds	50 mL

1. In a large bowl, stir together all-purpose flour, whole wheat flour, baking soda, baking powder, cinnamon, nutmeg, cloves and salt.

2. In a medium bowl, beat together egg, pumpkin purée, soy milk, brown sugar, pumpkin seeds, currants, oil and all but 1 tbsp (15 mL) sesame seeds. Using a fork, stir into dry ingredients just until moistened. Spoon into prepared muffin cups and sprinkle with the remaining sesame seeds.

3. Bake in preheated oven for 20 to 25 minutes, or until tops spring back when lightly touched.

Banana Bran Muffins with Cinnamon Sugar Topping

Serve one of these muffins with a Tofu Fruit Smoothie (see recipe, page 265) for a mini meal on the run.

TIP

To make cinnamon sugar, combine 2 tbsp (25 mL) packed brown sugar and 1 tsp (5 mL) ground cinnamon.

MAKE AHEAD

Place in an airtight container and store at room temperature for up to 2 days or in the freezer for up to 4 months.

Nutritional value
Per serving (1 muffin)

Calories	196
Protein	4 g
Fat	7 g
Carbohydrate	31 g
Dietary Fiber (a source)	2 g
Calcium	27 mg

Percent of calories from

Protein	8%
Fat	32%
Carbohydrate	60%

- Preheat oven to 375°F (190°C)
- 12-cup muffin tin, greased or lined with paper baking cups

1 cup	natural bran	250 mL
1 cup	all-purpose flour	250 mL
1/2 cup	whole wheat flour	125 mL
1 tsp	baking soda	5 mL
1 tsp	baking powder	5 mL
1/2 tsp	salt	2 mL
1/2 tsp	ground nutmeg	2 mL
3	large ripe bananas, mashed	3
2	eggs	2
1/2 cup	packed brown sugar	125 mL
1/3 cup	vegetable oil	75 mL
1 tsp	vanilla	5 mL
	Cinnamon sugar (see tip, at left)	

1. In a large bowl, stir together bran, all-purpose flour, whole wheat flour, baking soda, baking powder, salt and nutmeg.

2. In a medium bowl, beat together bananas, eggs, brown sugar, oil and vanilla. Using a fork, stir into dry ingredients just until moistened. Spoon into prepared muffin cups and sprinkle with cinnamon sugar.

3. Bake in preheated oven for 20 to 25 minutes, or until tops spring back when lightly touched.

Carrot, Apple and Almond Muffins

The ever-popular carrot muffin takes on a new guise in this lactose-free version. Applesauce keeps these muffins moist with a minimum of fat and adds a delicate flavor. Serve for breakfast, lunch or a nourishing coffee break.

MAKES 12 LARGE MUFFINS

TIP

For an appealing look, sprinkle a little grated carrot over batter before baking.

MAKE AHEAD

Place in an airtight container and store in the refrigerator for up to 1 week or in the freezer for up to 3 months.

Nutritional value
Per serving (1 muffin)

Calories	226
Protein	5 g
Fat	7 g
Carbohydrate	37 g
Dietary Fiber (a high source)	4 g
Calcium (a source)	58 mg

Percent of calories from

Protein	9%
Fat	28%
Carbohydrate	64%

* Preheat oven to 375°F (190°C)
* 12-cup muffin tin, greased or lined with paper baking cups

1 cup	whole wheat flour	250 mL
1 cup	all-purpose flour	250 mL
1 cup	lightly packed brown sugar	250 mL
2 tsp	ground cinnamon	10 mL
1 tsp	baking soda	5 mL
1 tsp	baking powder	5 mL
1/2 tsp	salt	2 mL
1/2 tsp	ground nutmeg	2 mL
2	eggs	2
2	large carrots, peeled and coarsely grated (2 1/4 cups/550 mL)	2
1 cup	unsweetened applesauce	250 mL
1/2 cup	toasted chopped almonds (see tip, page 195)	125 mL
1/4 cup	vegetable oil	50 mL

1. In a large bowl, stir together whole wheat flour, all-purpose flour, brown sugar, cinnamon, baking soda, baking powder, salt and nutmeg.

2. In a medium bowl, whisk together eggs, carrots, applesauce, almonds and oil. Using a fork, stir into dry ingredients just until moistened. Spoon into prepared muffin cups.

3. Bake in preheated oven for 20 to 25 minutes, or until tops spring back when lightly touched.

Desserts

For many people, life without dessert is like life without sunshine. Yet the world of dessert — puddings, cheesecakes, chocolate, ice cream — is a no-man's land for the lactose intolerant. This is dairy country. However, with careful substitutions, all of these delights can be enjoyed, as the recipes in this chapter demonstrate.

Cozy comfort desserts, including puddings, pies and crisps, which often include milk products and are served with milk, cream or ice cream, take on a new face when you use fruit juices and vegetable oils to replace the dairy. Likewise, silken tofu and drained yogurt can be used to replace the sour cream and cheese in the ever-popular cheesecake.

Of course, chocolate is a must for many dessert lovers. Although pure cocoa and chocolate are lactose-free, milk chocolate and many chocolate by-products are not. The recipes here demonstrate the ease of cooking with cocoa and pure chocolate to create that richness so desirable to the chocolate lover.

For many, a life without ice cream is unimaginable! A luscious ending to a rich meal or a cooling slurp on a hot day, ice cream is one of life's simple pleasures. Although traditional ice cream made with a rich cream custard is definitely off the menu, frozen soufflé versions made with beaten egg white and fresh sorbets made with fruit purées are grand finales with no lactose.

Taste for yourself and enjoy these scrumptious lactose-free desserts!

Basic Custard 207	Pumpkin Pie 218
Sesame Crunch 208	Basic Sponge Cake 220
Dried Fruit Compote 209	Caramelized Peach Rice Gâteau 222
Fruited Truffles 210	Fudge Cake 223
Bread Pudding 211	Lemon Cheesecake 224
Creamy Stovetop Rice Pudding 212	Amaretto Cheesecake 225
Cappuccino Cookies 213	Raspberry Cheesecake in a Glass . . . 226
Shortbread 214	Chocolate Cheesecake Squares 227
Basic Meringue 215	Drained Yogurt Cheesecake 228
Oatmeal Shortbread with Date Filling 216	Tiramisu 230

(continued on next page…)

Fudge Pudding 232

Chocolate Mousse 234

Biscuit Tortoni 235

Vanilla Ice Cream. 236

Mango Sorbet. 238

Banana Sorbet 239

Apricot Sorbet. 240

Basic Custard

Custard is one of the original comfort foods. When made with milk, it is considered a calcium-rich dessert that's nutritious for children. But there is nothing to say custard has to be made with milk (although that version is below). Try any variety of juices, even coffee, for a wonderful sauce over fruit or cake or in a trifle.

MAKES ABOUT 1½ CUPS (375 ML) OR 4 SERVINGS

4	egg yolks	4
½ cup	granulated sugar	125 mL
1 cup	fortified orange juice	250 mL

1. In a heavy stainless steel saucepan, whisk together egg yolks and sugar until smooth. Gradually whisk in orange juice. Cook over medium heat, whisking frequently to prevent curdling, until thickened, about 5 minutes.

Variation

Lactose-Free Custard: For a milk-based custard, substitute lactose-free milk or fortified soy milk for the orange juice; add 1 tsp (5 mL) vanilla.

Nutritional value
Per serving

Calories	182
Protein	3 g
Fat	5 g
Carbohydrate	32 g
Dietary Fiber	0 g
Calcium	29 mg

Percent of calories from

Protein	7%
Fat	25%
Carbohydrate	68%

Sesame Crunch

An ideal lunchtime treat, this square packs a powerful calcium punch from sesame seeds and almonds. It's a fun recipe for children to help with, especially when they can mix the ingredients with their hands.

MAKES ABOUT 30 SQUARES

TIP

Toasting nuts and seeds intensifies their flavor. To toast almonds and sesame seeds, bake in preheated 350°F (180°C) oven for 10 to 12 minutes, or until golden brown and fragrant.

- Preheat oven to 350°F (180°C)
- 8-inch (2 L) square baking dish, greased or sprayed with nonstick baking spray

2 cups	corn flakes cereal	500 mL
1 cup	quick-cooking rolled oats	250 mL
1/2 cup	chopped toasted almonds (see tip, at left)	125 mL
1/2 cup	toasted sesame seeds (see tip, at left)	125 mL
1/2 cup	liquid honey	125 mL
1/2 cup	packed brown sugar	125 mL

1. In a large bowl, using your hands or the base of small bowl, crush corn flakes to coarse crumbs. Stir in oats, almonds, sesame seeds, honey and brown sugar until well combined. Pack firmly into prepared baking dish.

2. Bake in preheated oven for 25 minutes, or until golden brown. While still warm, cut into squares with a sharp knife. Let cool completely before removing from pan.

Nutritional value
Per serving (1 square)

Calories	73
Protein	2 g
Fat	3 g
Carbohydrate	12 g
Dietary Fiber	1 g
Calcium	37 mg

Percent of calories from

Protein	8%
Fat	29%
Carbohydrate	63%

Dried Fruit Compote

Wonderful for breakfast or a winter dessert, the dried fruits are a source of calcium. Be sure to use orange juice fortified with calcium and vitamin D to boost your calcium intake.

TIP

This fruit salad tastes better when it has a chance to mellow overnight in the refrigerator.

1 cup	halved dried figs	250 mL
1 cup	halved dried apricots	250 mL
1 cup	halved dried prunes or dates	250 mL
1	slice lemon peel	1
1	cinnamon stick	1
2 cups	fortified orange juice	500 mL
1/4 cup	granulated sugar	50 mL
1/3 cup	chopped toasted almonds (see tip, page 208)	75 mL
	Basic Custard Sauce (see recipe, page 262) (optional)	

1. In a medium bowl, cover figs, apricots and prunes with boiling water. Let stand for at least 5 minutes, until plump. Drain.

2. In a large saucepan, combine fruit mixture, lemon peel, cinnamon stick, orange juice and sugar. Bring to a boil over medium-high heat; reduce heat to medium and simmer, uncovered, until fruit is very plump, about 5 minutes. Transfer to a bowl, cover and refrigerate for at least 4 hours, until chilled, or overnight.

3. Serve in small glass dishes, sprinkled with almonds and Basic Custard Sauce, if desired.

Variations

Add the grated zest of one lemon to fruit mixture.

Use one or two dried fruits instead of three; just make sure the total quantity equals 3 cups (750 mL).

Nutritional value
Per serving

Calories	226
Protein	3 g
Fat	4 g
Carbohydrate	49 g
Dietary Fiber (a very high source)	6 g
Calcium (a source)	160 mg

Percent of calories from

Protein	5%
Fat	14%
Carbohydrate	81%

Fruited Truffles

These self-righteous truffles are calcium-enhanced, low in fat and lactose-free.

MAKES ABOUT 30 TRUFFLES

TIP

Toasting nuts intensifies their flavor. To toast almonds, bake in preheated 350°F (180°C) oven for 10 to 12 minutes, or until golden brown and fragrant.

MAKE AHEAD

Place in an airtight container and store in the refrigerator for up to 1 week or in the freezer for up to 3 months.

1 cup	chopped dried figs, hard stems removed	250 mL
1 cup	chopped dried apricots	250 mL
1 cup	toasted chopped almonds (see tip, at left)	250 mL
1 tbsp	grated orange zest	15 mL
2 tbsp	fortified orange juice	25 mL
2 tbsp	granulated sugar	25 mL

1. In a food processor, using pulsing action, chop figs, apricots and almonds until finely chopped. Add orange zest and orange juice and process until well combined.

2. Place sugar in a small bowl. Form 1 tbsp (15 mL) of the fruit mixture into a ball and roll in sugar to coat. Repeat with remaining mixture to make about 30 truffles.

Nutritional value
Per serving (1 truffle)

Calories	56
Protein	1 g
Fat	2 g
Carbohydrate	9 g
Dietary Fiber (a source)	2 g
Calcium	24 mg

Percent of calories from

Protein	9%
Fat	34%
Carbohydrate	58%

Bread Pudding

This dressed-up version of a popular classic has a fanciful meringue topping that makes it special enough to serve to guests as well as family.

- Preheat oven to 350°F (180°C)
- 12-cup (3 L) baking dish, greased

¾ cup	raisins	175 mL
6 cups	cubed bread (about 8 slices)	1.5 L
3 cups	lactose-free milk or fortified soy milk	750 mL
4	egg yolks	4
½ cup	packed brown sugar	125 mL
1 tsp	ground cinnamon	5 mL
1 tsp	vanilla	5 mL
¼ tsp	salt	1 mL
¼ tsp	ground nutmeg	1 mL

Topping

4	egg whites	4
Pinch	salt	Pinch
¼ cup	granulated sugar	50 mL
1 tsp	vanilla	5 mL
2 tbsp	toasted chopped almonds	25 mL

Basic Custard (see recipe, page 207)

1. In a small bowl, pour boiling water over raisins. In a large bowl, stir together bread, milk, egg yolks, brown sugar, cinnamon, vanilla, salt and nutmeg. Drain raisins and stir into bread mixture.

2. *Prepare the topping:* In a clean bowl, using an electric mixer, beat egg whites and salt on high speed until soft peaks form. Gradually beat in sugar and vanilla until stiff peaks form.

3. Spoon bread mixture into prepared baking dish. Spread meringue evenly over top, making decorative swirls with a knife. Sprinkle with almonds.

4. Bake in preheated oven for 50 to 60 minutes, or until meringue is golden brown and bread seems moist but set. Serve with Basic Custard.

Nutritional value
Per serving (without Basic Custard)

Calories	324
Protein	10 g
Fat	7 g
Carbohydrate	57 g
Dietary Fiber	1 g
Calcium (a high source)	174 mg

Percent of calories from

Protein	12%
Fat	19%
Carbohydrate	69%

Creamy Stovetop Rice Pudding

It's hard to believe that a dessert so good can be nutritious too! In fact, it's so healthy, you could eat it for breakfast.

TIPS

The creaminess in this rice pudding comes from a combination of short-grain rice, fruit juice and egg to give it a custard-like texture and smooth taste.

Italian short-grain rice, available in supermarkets, works well in this dessert.

3 cups	water, divided	750 mL
1	cinnamon stick	1
1/2 cup	short-grain rice	125 mL
1 cup	apple juice	250 mL
1/3 cup	loosely packed brown sugar	75 mL
1 tsp	vanilla	5 mL
1/4 tsp	ground nutmeg	1 mL
2	eggs, beaten	2
1/3 cup	currants, washed, or raisins	75 mL

1. In a large saucepan, bring 2 cups (500 mL) of the water and cinnamon stick to a boil over high heat. Stir in rice and return to a boil; reduce heat to low, cover and simmer for 35 to 40 minutes, or until rice is very tender and water has been absorbed.

2. Stir in the remaining 1 cup (250 mL) water, apple juice, brown sugar, vanilla and nutmeg. Cook, covered, over low heat until rice is creamy, about 10 minutes.

3. Beat in eggs and currants. Cook, stirring, until thickened and creamy, about 2 minutes. Discard cinnamon stick. For best flavor, serve warm.

Variation

For an extra calcium punch, try making this pudding with fortified orange juice instead of apple juice.

Nutritional value
Per serving

Calories	160
Protein	3 g
Fat	2 g
Carbohydrate	32 g
Dietary Fiber	1 g
Calcium	32 mg

Percent of calories from

Protein	8%
Fat	12%
Carbohydrate	81%

Cappuccino Cookies

Originally, these were a buttery shortbread-like cookie, but shortening and added flavoring make a good substitute for butter to produce a melt-in-your-mouth cookie that's rich in flavor.

MAKE AHEAD

Store raw dough in an airtight container in the freezer for up to 2 months. Store baked cookies in an airtight container in the freezer for up to 4 months.

Nutritional value
Per serving (1 cookie)

Calories	97
Protein	1 g
Fat	5 g
Carbohydrate	14 g
Dietary Fiber	0 g
Calcium	7 mg

Percent of calories from

Protein	3%
Fat	42%
Carbohydrate	54%

- Preheat oven to 350°F (180°C)
- Baking sheet, lined with parchment paper

2½ cups	cake-and-pastry flour	625 mL
½ cup	unsweetened cocoa powder	125 mL
1 tsp	ground cinnamon	5 mL
½ tsp	salt	2 mL
1 tbsp	instant coffee granules	15 mL
1 tbsp	vanilla	15 mL
1	egg	1
1 cup	granulated sugar, divided	250 mL
1 cup	packed brown sugar	250 mL
1 cup	shortening	250 mL

1. In a medium bowl, stir together flour, cocoa, cinnamon and salt; set aside.

2. In a small bowl, dissolve coffee in vanilla; set aside.

3. In a large bowl, using an electric mixer, beat together egg, ¾ cup (175 mL) of the granulated sugar, brown sugar and shortening until fluffy. Gradually beat in flour mixture and coffee mixture until dough starts to hold together.

4. Divide mixture into 48 equal portions and form into 1-inch (2.5 cm) balls. Place the remaining granulated sugar in a small bowl and roll each ball in sugar to coat.

5. Arrange cookies on prepared baking sheet, leaving 1 inch (2.5 cm) between each. Bake in batches in preheated oven for about 20 minutes, or until firm to the touch.

Shortbread

Shortbread relies upon the unique flavor of butter for its magnificence. This lactose-free version uses shortening for texture and brown sugar and vanilla for flavor. Taste these to see if they don't measure up to the traditional cookie!

MAKES ABOUT 4 DOZEN

TIP

Parchment (or silicone) paper makes removing baked goods from baking pans easy. It is available in many supermarkets and cookery stores.

● *Preheat oven to 350°F (180°C)*
● *Baking sheet, lined with parchment paper*

2 cups	all-purpose flour	500 mL
1/2 cup	rice flour	125 mL
1/2 tsp	salt	2 mL
1 cup	shortening	250 mL
2/3 cup	packed brown sugar	150 mL
2 tsp	vanilla	10 mL

1. In a medium bowl, stir together all-purpose flour, rice flour and salt.

2. In a large bowl, using an electric mixer, beat together shortening, brown sugar and vanilla until fluffy. Gradually beat in flour mixture, 1/2 cup (125 mL) at a time, scraping down bowl occasionally.

3. Roll dough out between 2 sheets of waxed paper to 1/4-inch (5 mm) thickness. Remove top layer of paper. Using a fancy cookie cutter, cut out cookies and arrange on prepared baking sheet. Re-roll dough and continue to cut out until all dough is used.

4. Bake in preheated oven for 20 to 25 minutes, or until golden brown.

Nutritional value
Per serving (1 shortbread)

Calories	72
Protein	1 g
Fat	4 g
Carbohydrate	8 g
Dietary Fiber	0 g
Calcium	3 mg

Percent of calories from

Protein	4%
Fat	54%
Carbohydrate	42%

Basic Meringue

Here's another lactose-free, lower-fat recipe that can take many guises. Serve small meringues piled in a glass bowl drizzled with Cappuccino Sauce (see recipe, page 260) or make the dessert meringues and fill with a spoonful of Lemon Butter (see recipe, page 255) and top with sliced strawberries. Or make into layers and spread with Lemon Butter, sprinkle with sliced berries and stack for a torte.

MAKES 24 SMALL OR 8 DESSERT MERINGUES, OR 3 TORTE LAYERS

MAKE AHEAD

Place in a dry airtight container, such as a cake tin, and store at room temperature for up to 1 week or in the freezer for up to 4 months. Do not store in plastic or meringue will become soft.

Nutritional value
Per Serving (¹/₂₄th of recipe)

Calories	35
Protein	1 g
Fat	0 g
Carbohydrate	8 g
Dietary Fiber	0 g
Calcium	0 mg

Percent of calories from

Protein	6%
Fat	0%
Carbohydrate	94%

- *Preheat oven to 300°F (150°C)*
- *Baking sheet, lined with parchment paper*

4	egg whites	4
½ tsp	cream of tartar	2 mL
1 cup	granulated sugar	250 mL
1 tsp	vanilla	5 mL

1. In a medium bowl, using an electric mixer, beat egg whites and cream of tartar on high speed until soft peaks form. Gradually beat in sugar, 1 tablespoonful (15 mL) at a time, until stiff peaks form. Fold in vanilla.

2. *For small meringues,* spoon by heaped teaspoons (5 mL) onto baking sheet lined with parchment paper, forming into peaks and leaving 2 inches (5 cm) between each. *For dessert meringues,* spoon about ¼ cup (50 mL) for each meringue onto baking sheet, leaving 2 inches (5 cm) between each; using the back of a dampened spoon, indent centers. *For torte layers,* using a 9-inch (23 cm) plate as a template, draw 3 circles on parchment. Spread even quantities of meringue onto circles, leaving a 1-inch (2.5 cm) border uncovered.

3. In preheated oven, bake small meringues or torte layers for 25 to 30 minutes, large meringues for 30 to 35 minutes, or until golden brown. Turn oven off and let cool completely in oven.

Oatmeal Shortbread with Date Filling

This is the sort of cookie my grandmother would have made. She would not have known the cookie was lactose-free and the date filling was a calcium source. But everyone knew it was tasty and the perfect addition to a lunch-bag.

MAKES 2 DOZEN COOKIES

TIPS

Dipping your knife or scissors blade in hot water will make it easier to cut the sticky dates.

Dates, figs and apricots are all sources of calcium. Figs have the most, with 120 mg per ½ cup (125 mL), while dates and apricots have 30 mg per ½ cup (125 mL).

- Preheat oven to 325°F (160°C)
- Baking sheet, lined with parchment paper
- 2-inch (10 cm) round cookie cutter

2½ cups	cake and pastry flour	625 mL
1 tsp	baking soda	5 mL
1 tsp	salt	5 mL
1 cup	packed brown sugar	250 mL
1 cup	shortening	250 mL
½ cup	lactose-free milk	125 mL
1 tsp	vinegar	5 mL
2½ cups	quick-cooking rolled oats	625 mL

Date Filling

8 oz	pitted dates	250 g
1 cup	water	250 mL
¼ cup	granulated sugar	50 mL
1 tbsp	grated orange zest	15 mL

1. In a medium bowl, sift together flour, baking soda and salt.

2. In a large bowl, cream brown sugar and shortening until fluffy.

3. In a measuring cup, combine milk and vinegar. Let stand for 5 minutes.

4. Using a wooden spoon or an electric mixer, beat flour mixture, milk mixture and oats into creamed mixture until well combined. Form into a ball.

Nutritional value
Per serving (1 cookie)

Calories	232
Protein	3 g
Fat	10 g
Carbohydrate	34 g
Dietary Fiber (a source)	2 g
Calcium	25 mg

Percent of calories from

Protein	5%
Fat	37%
Carbohydrate	58%

5. Roll dough out between 2 layers of waxed paper to ¼-inch (0.5 cm) thickness. Cut out with cookie cutter and place on baking sheet.

6. Bake in preheated oven for 12 to 15 minutes, or until golden brown. Let cool on wire racks.

7. *Meanwhile, prepare the filling:* Using a sharp knife, cut dates; place in a medium saucepan. Add water, sugar and orange zest. Bring to a boil over medium heat and cook until dates are soft, about 5 minutes. Let cool.

8. Spread a heaped teaspoonful (5 mL) of date filling on the smooth side of one cookie; place another cookie on top. Repeat until all cookies are used.

Variation

Chopped figs and/or apricots can be used to replace some or all of the dates.

MAKE AHEAD

Place unfilled cookies in airtight containers and store at room temperature for up to 3 days. Once spread with date filling, place cookies in airtight containers and store in the freezer for up to 4 months.

Pumpkin Pie

Serve this with Yogurt Sauce (see recipe, page 250) or Vanilla Ice Cream (see recipe, page 230) for a traditional harvest dessert.

MAKES 6 SERVINGS

TIP

Rolling out pastry is often a dreaded task for even the best bakers. Try this foolproof method to simplify pastry making. With a rolling pin, roll pastry out between 2 sheets of waxed paper, rolling away from your body and holding the waxed paper firmly between the counter and your stomach. Turn paper as needed to form pastry into circle. Gently remove top layer of waxed paper; replace. Flip over and remove other piece of paper. Invert 9-inch

Nutritional value
Per serving

Calories	261
Protein	4 g
Fat	10 g
Carbohydrate	37 g
Dietary Fiber (a source)	2 g
Calcium	44 mg

Percent of calories from

Protein	6%
Fat	34%
Carbohydrate	56%

● *Preheat oven to 425°F (220°C)*
● *9-inch (23 cm) pie plate*

Crust

1 cup	all-purpose flour	250 mL
1/4 tsp	salt	1 mL
1/3 cup	shortening (at room temperature)	75 mL
3 tbsp	cold water	50 mL

Filling

2	eggs	2
1	can (14 oz/398 mL) pumpkin purée (not pie filling)	1
1 cup	fortified soy milk or lactose-free milk	250 mL
3/4 cup	loosely packed brown sugar	175 mL
2 tbsp	dark rum	25 mL
2 tbsp	liquid honey	25 mL
1 tsp	ground cinnamon	5 mL
1 tsp	ground ginger	5 mL
1/2 tsp	ground cloves	2 mL
1/4 tsp	ground nutmeg	1 mL
1/4 tsp	salt	1 mL

1. *Prepare the crust:* In a medium bowl, stir together flour and salt. Using a pastry blender or 2 knives, cut in shortening until mixture resembles coarse crumbs. Using a fork, stir in water just until pastry sticks together. Form into a ball.

2. Roll out pastry and fit into pie plate (see tip, at left).

3. *Prepare the filling:* In a large bowl, whisk together eggs, pumpkin purée, milk, brown sugar, rum, honey, cinnamon, ginger, cloves, nutmeg and salt. Pour into crust.

4. Bake in preheated oven for 20 to 25 minutes, or until golden brown. Reduce heat to 350°F (180°C) and continue to bake for 25 to 30 minutes, or until firm. Let cool.

(23 cm) pie plate onto pastry and flip. Gently remove remaining waxed paper. Ease pastry into pie plate, letting it relax against sides. Crimp edges and set aside.

Basic Sponge Cake

This is one of the easiest, most versatile lactose-free cake recipes that bakers can have in their repertoire. Depending on the shape of pan used, you have a different creation. Every winter I use it as a jelly roll for the traditional Yule Log. Each spring it is transformed with the addition of lemon zest, lemon filling and a sprinkling of strawberries. The variations are endless, as you will discover when you start concocting your own.

MAKES 1 CAKE OR JELLY ROLL

TIPS

You can also use this recipe to make a layer cake. Fill it with raspberry jam and sprinkle it with confectioner's sugar for an everyday treat.

Always check eggs before using. Discard any with cracked shells, as they may carry the salmonella bacteria.

3	eggs	3
1 cup	granulated sugar	250 mL
1/3 cup	water	75 mL
1 tsp	vanilla	5 mL
1 cup	all-purpose flour	250 mL
1 tsp	baking powder	5 mL
1/4 tsp	salt	1 mL
	Confectioner's (icing) sugar (for jelly roll only)	

Cake

1. Preheat oven to 350°F (180°C). Line the bottom of a 9-inch (23 cm) round cake pan with waxed paper.

2. In a medium bowl, using an electric mixer, beat eggs on high speed until light in color. Gradually beat in sugar until thick and pale-colored. Beat in water and vanilla.

3. Sift flour, baking powder and salt over egg mixture; beat until combined. Pour into prepared pan.

4. Bake for 25 to 30 minutes, or until golden brown. Let stand for 10 minutes before inverting onto a wire rack and removing waxed paper.

Jelly Roll

1. Preheat oven to 375°F (190°C). Line the bottom of a 15- by 10-inch (38 by 25 cm) jelly-roll pan with waxed paper.

2. In a medium bowl, using an electric mixer, beat eggs on high speed until light in color. Gradually beat in sugar until thick and pale-colored. Beat in water and vanilla.

3. Sift flour, baking powder and salt over egg mixture; beat until combined. Pour into prepared pan.

Nutritional value
Per serving (1/8th of recipe)

Calories	184
Protein	4 g
Fat	2 g
Carbohydrate	37 g
Dietary Fiber	1 g
Calcium	20 mg

Percent of calories from

Protein	8%
Fat	11%
Carbohydrate	81%

4. Bake for 15 to 20 minutes, or until golden brown. Let stand for 10 minutes. Sift confectioner's sugar over a clean tea towel. Invert pan over towel. Remove pan and gently remove waxed paper. Roll up jelly roll along short end in tea towel. Cool completely. Unroll and remove towel to fill.

Variations

Apple Jelly Roll or Sponge Layer Cake: Substitute apple juice for water and add $1/2$ tsp (2 mL) ground cinnamon. Fill with Apple Butter (see recipe, page 254) and sift confectioner's sugar over surface. Decorate with apple slices dipped in lemon juice.

Citrus Jelly Roll or Sponge Layer Cake: Substitute fortified orange juice for water and add 1 tbsp (15 mL) grated lemon zest and 1 tbsp (15 mL) grated orange zest. Fill with Lemon or Lime Butter (see recipe and variation, page 255) and use it to pipe lemon rosettes onto surface. Garnish with kiwi or strawberries.

Chocolate Jelly Roll or Sponge Layer Cake: Reduce flour to $3/4$ cup (175 mL) and add $1/4$ cup (50 mL) unsweetened cocoa powder. Fill with Chocolate Cream Filling (see variation, page 258) and spread with Cappuccino Sauce (see recipe, page 260).

Yule Log: Unroll Chocolate Jelly Roll and spread with Coffee Cream Filling (see variation, page 258), re-roll. Trim ends at an angle; place cut pieces on top of either end of the "log" as "knots." Spread outside of log with thin layer of Cappuccino Sauce (see recipe, page 260). Dab remaining coffee filling at the end and on top of knots for "snow." Carefully transfer to serving platter and garnish base with fresh greenery from evergreen.

Yule Log: Nutritional value Per Serving (⅛th of recipe)

Calories: 443, Protein: 16 g, Fat: 9 g, Carbohydrate: 81 g, Dietary Fiber: 3 g (a source), Calcium: 71 mg (a source)

Percent of calories from
Protein: 13%, Fat: 18%, Carbohydrate: 68%

MAKE AHEAD

Let cake or jelly roll cool completely, wrap in plastic wrap, then foil, and store in the freezer for up to 4 months.

Caramelized Peach Rice Gâteau

Although this is supposed to serve six, I must admit to polishing off more than my generous share! For lovers of rice pudding, this chic version is certainly worth making for guests. It should be served at room temperature with a garnish of sliced peaches and a sprig of mint.

MAKES 6 SERVINGS

TIP

Peach cocktail is a peach drink made from a variety of fruit juices and peach purée with a delicate taste that says "peach." It is available in the juice section of grocery stores.

MAKE AHEAD

Can be prepared through Step 3, covered and stored in the refrigerator for up to 4 hours.

Nutritional value
Per serving

Calories	191
Protein	4 g
Fat	4 g
Carbohydrate	37 g
Dietary Fiber	1 g
Calcium	30 mg

Percent of calories from

Protein	7%
Fat	16%
Carbohydrate	77%

- Preheat oven to 350°F (180°C)
- 6-cup (1.5 L) shallow baking dish, greased

2 cups	water	500 mL
½ cup	short-grain rice	125 mL
2	eggs, beaten	2
1 cup	peach cocktail (see tip, at left)	250 mL
½ cup	granulated sugar	125 mL
1 tsp	grated lemon zest	5 mL
½ tsp	almond extract	2 mL
¼ tsp	ground nutmeg	1 mL
2 tbsp	chopped toasted almonds	25 mL
2 tbsp	packed brown sugar	25 mL

1. In a medium saucepan, bring water to a boil over high heat. Stir in rice and return to a boil; reduce heat to low, cover and simmer for 35 to 40 minutes, or until rice is very tender and water has been absorbed.

2. In a large bowl, whisk together eggs, peach cocktail, sugar, lemon zest, almond extract and nutmeg. Gradually whisk in cooked rice. Pour into prepared baking dish.

3. Bake, uncovered, in preheated oven for 55 to 60 minutes, or until set. Mixture will jiggle in center but will firm up on cooling. Let stand for 1 hour.

4. Sprinkle top evenly with almonds and brown sugar. Broil until sugar has caramelized, about 2 minutes. Serve at once.

> Short-grain rice is used for desserts to give a creamy pudding texture, one that sticks together. Long-grain rice tends to be more separate and, as such, is ideal for rice pilafs.

Fudge Cake

Birthdays in our house would not be complete without this cake. Spread with Cappuccino Sauce (see recipe, page 260) and serve with an accompanying bowl of sauce for both the cake and one of the ice creams (see recipes, pages 236–37). It's a winning combination.

MAKES 12 SERVINGS

MAKE AHEAD

Wrap cake in plastic wrap, then in aluminum foil, and store in the freezer for up to 4 months. (Wrap it well so no one knows what's inside!)

Nutritional value
Per serving (without sauce)

Calories	379
Protein	6 g
Fat	15 g
Carbohydrate	60 g
Dietary Fiber	1 g
Calcium (a source)	41 mg

Percent of calories from

Protein	6%
Fat	34%
Carbohydrate	60%

- Preheat oven to 350°F (180°C)
- 9-inch (23 cm) springform pan, lined with parchment paper

2 cups	all-purpose flour	500 mL
3/4 cup	unsweetened cocoa powder	175 mL
2 tsp	baking powder	10 mL
1 tsp	baking soda	5 mL
1 tsp	ground cinnamon	5 mL
1/2 tsp	salt	2 mL
1 1/2 cups	granulated sugar	375 mL
3/4 cup	shortening	175 mL
3	eggs	3
1 tbsp	instant coffee granules	15 mL
1 1/4 cups	warm water	300 mL
1 tsp	vanilla	5 mL

1. In a medium bowl, sift together flour, cocoa, baking powder, baking soda, cinnamon and salt.

2. In another large bowl, using an electric mixer, beat sugar and shortening until fluffy. Beat in eggs, one at a time, until well combined.

3. Dissolve coffee in warm water.

4. Beat flour mixture and coffee alternately into shortening mixture, making 2 additions of dry and 1 of wet. Stir in vanilla. Spoon evenly into prepared pan.

5. Bake in preheated oven for 55 to 65 minutes, or until tester inserted in centre comes out clean. Let cool in pan on a wire rack for 10 minutes. Run a knife around edge of pan; remove cake and discard paper. Let cool completely on rack.

Lemon Cheesecake

One of my favorite desserts, this New York–style cheesecake uses tofu to replace the usual cream cheese. Try it with a spoonful of Quick Strawberry or Blueberry Sauce (see recipe and variation, page 259).

(see recipe and variation, page 259).

MAKES 8 SERVINGS

Nutritional value
Per serving

Calories	357
Protein	9 g
Fat	13 g
Carbohydrate	53 g
Dietary Fiber	0 g
Calcium	47 mg

Percent of calories from

Protein	10%
Fat	31%
Carbohydrate	59%

- Preheat oven to 350°F (180°C)
- 9-inch (23 cm) springform pan

Crust

1 1/2 cups	graham wafer crumbs	375 mL
1/4 cup	granulated sugar	50 mL
3 tbsp	vegetable oil	45 mL
1 tsp	ground cinnamon	5 mL

Filling

2	packages (each 10 1/4 oz/297 g) silken firm tofu	2
4	eggs, separated	4
1 cup	granulated sugar	250 mL
1 tbsp	grated lemon zest	15 mL
1/4 cup	freshly squeezed lemon juice	50 mL
2 tbsp	all-purpose flour	25 mL
1 tsp	vanilla	5 mL
1/2 tsp	salt	2 mL

1. *Prepare the crust:* In a small mixing bowl, stir together graham wafer crumbs, sugar, oil and cinnamon. Press onto bottom and 1 inch (2.5 cm) up sides of pan. Bake in preheated oven for 10 minutes. Let cool.

2. *Meanwhile, prepare the filling:* Using a sieve, drain tofu. In a food processor, beat together drained tofu, egg yolks, sugar, lemon zest, lemon juice, flour, vanilla and salt until smooth.

3. In a clean bowl, using an electric mixer, beat egg whites on high speed until stiff peaks form. Fold into lemon mixture. Turn into prepared crust.

4. Bake for 60 to 65 minutes, or until almost firm in center. Let cool before cutting into wedges to serve.

Amaretto Cheesecake

Silken firm tofu makes a good substitute for cream cheese in this delicate almond cheesecake. It may be made up to 1 day ahead.

MAKES 8 SERVINGS

TIP

Toasting nuts intensifies their flavor. To toast almonds, bake in preheated 350°F (180°C) oven for 10 to 12 minutes, or until golden brown and fragrant.

MAKE AHEAD

Wrap cake in plastic wrap and store in the refrigerator for up to 4 hours.

Nutritional value

Per serving

Calories	308
Protein	9 g
Fat	13 g
Carbohydrate	37 g
Dietary Fiber	1 g
Calcium	68 mg
(a source)	

Percent of calories from

Protein	12%
Fat	37%
Carbohydrate	46%

- Preheat oven to 350°F (180°C)
- 10-inch (25 cm) pie plate, sprayed with nonstick baking spray

Crust

1 cup	vanilla wafer crumbs	250 mL
¼ cup	granulated sugar	50 mL
¼ cup	toasted sliced almonds (see tip, at left)	50 mL
2 tbsp	vegetable oil	25 mL
¼ tsp	almond extract	1 mL

Filling

2	packages (each 10.25 oz/297 g) silken firm tofu	2
2	eggs	2
½ cup	granulated sugar	125 mL
⅓ cup	amaretto liqueur	75 mL
1 tsp	grated lemon zest	5 mL
¼ cup	sliced almonds	50 mL

1. *Prepare the crust:* In a small mixing bowl, stir together vanilla wafer crumbs, sugar, almonds, oil and almond extract. Press onto bottom and up side of prepared pie plate.

2. *Meanwhile, prepare the filling:* Using a sieve, drain tofu. In a food processor, purée drained tofu, eggs, sugar, amaretto and lemon zest until smooth. Pour into prepared crust. Sprinkle almonds on surface around edge.

3. Bake in preheated oven for 50 to 55 minutes, or until firm.

Raspberry Cheesecake in a Glass

Similar to a Bavarian cream but lower in fat than the traditional one made with whipping cream, this tofu version has a full, rich fruit flavor once it is well chilled and set.

3	packages (each 10.25 oz/290 g) silken soft tofu	3
1	envelope (1/4 oz/7 g) unflavored gelatin	1
1	can (10 oz/300 mL) undiluted raspberry juice concentrate, divided	1
1/3 cup	granulated sugar	75 mL
2 tsp	vanilla	10 mL
	Fresh raspberries	

1. Using a sieve, drain tofu.

2. In a small saucepan, sprinkle gelatin over 1/2 cup (125 mL) of the raspberry concentrate. Let stand for 10 minutes. Heat over low heat, stirring, for 2 to 3 minutes, or until gelatin dissolves.

3. In a food processor, purée drained tofu, the remaining raspberry concentrate, sugar and vanilla until smooth. With motor running, pour in dissolved gelatin through feed tube. Purée until well combined.

4. Pour about 1/2-cup (125 mL) servings into dainty serving bowls. Cover and refrigerate for at least 4 hours. Serve with a sprinkling of fresh raspberries.

Nutritional value
Per serving

Calories	98
Protein	5 g
Fat	3 g
Carbohydrate	14 g
Dietary Fiber	0 g
Calcium	28 mg

Percent of calories from

Protein	20%
Fat	24%
Carbohydrate	57%

Chocolate Cheesecake Squares

Individual pieces can be picked up and enjoyed with a good cup of coffee.

MAKES 16 SQUARES

- Preheat oven to 350°F (180°C)
- 8-inch (2 L) square cake pan, lined with parchment paper

1 cup	graham wafer crumbs	250 mL
2 tbsp	granulated sugar	25 mL
2 tbsp	vegetable oil	25 mL
1/2 tsp	ground cinnamon	2 mL

Chocolate Filling

1	package (10.25 oz/290 g) silken soft tofu	1
2	eggs	2
2/3 cup	granulated sugar	175 mL
1/3 cup	unsweetened cocoa powder	75 mL
2 tsp	vanilla	10 mL
1/2 tsp	salt	2 mL
	Sliced strawberries (optional)	

1. In a small bowl, stir together graham wafer crumbs, sugar, oil and cinnamon. Press onto bottom of prepared pan.

2. Using a sieve, drain tofu. In a medium bowl, using an electric mixer, beat together drained tofu, eggs, sugar, cocoa, vanilla and salt until smooth. Pour into pan.

3. Bake in preheated oven for 35 to 40 minutes, or until firm. Let cool on a wire rack. Cut into 16 squares and garnish each piece with strawberry slice (if using).

Nutritional value
Per serving (1 square)

Calories	107
Protein	2 g
Fat	4 g
Carbohydrate	16 g
Dietary Fiber	0 g
Calcium	14 mg

Percent of calories from

Protein	8%
Fat	32%
Carbohydrate	59%

Drained Yogurt Cheesecake

For those who can digest yogurt, this no-bake cheesecake is the answer. It is bursting with flavor and calcium. If regular yogurt is a problem for you, try the lactose-free yogurts now available in grocery stores.

TIPS

Many people with lactose intolerance find that they can digest yogurt with natural bacteria. The bacteria help break down the lactose. If you can digest yogurt, try to incorporate it into your diet as a calcium source.

Garnish with slivers of apricots and fresh mint sprigs.

Nutritional value	
Per serving	
Calories	278
Protein	6 g
Fat	10 g
Carbohydrate	44 g
Dietary Fiber (a source)	2 g
Calcium (a source)	144 mg
Percent of calories from	
Protein	9%
Fat	30%
Carbohydrate	61%

- Preheat oven to 350°F (180°C)
- 9-inch (23 cm) springform pan, sprayed with baking spray

Crust

1 cup	graham cracker crumbs (about 15 squares)	250 mL
¼ cup	ground almonds	50 mL
¼ cup	vegetable oil	50 mL
2 tbsp	granulated sugar	25 mL
1 tsp	ground cinnamon	5 mL

Filling

1	container (26 oz/750 g) plain yogurt	1
2 cups	mixed dried fruit, such as figs, apricots and dates	500 mL
½ cup	granulated sugar	125 mL
1 tbsp	grated lemon zest	15 mL
¼ cup	freshly squeezed lemon juice	50 mL

1. *Prepare the crust:* In a small bowl, stir together graham cracker crumbs, almonds, oil, sugar and cinnamon. Press into prepared pan. Bake in preheated oven for 10 minutes, until golden brown. Let cool on a wire rack.

2. *Prepare the filling:* Spoon yogurt into a paper towel–lined sieve placed over a bowl. Cover, place in the refrigerator and let drain for at least 1 hour or overnight. You should end up with 2 cups (500 mL) yogurt and 1 cup (250 mL) liquid.

3. In a medium bowl, cover dried fruit with boiling water; let stand for 5 minutes, until soft and plump. Drain and coarsely chop. If using figs, remove tough stems.

4. In a food processor, using pulsing action, chop dried fruit, sugar, lemon zest and lemon juice until fruit is finely chopped. Transfer to a bowl and stir in drained yogurt.

5. Spoon filling into prepared crust. Cover and refrigerate for at least 1 hour, until chilled. Cut into wedges.

Variation

Use only two dried fruits, such as apricots and dates.

MAKE AHEAD

Store in the refrigerator for up to 1 day.

Tiramisu

The Italian version of trifle, tiramisu is typically made with a high-fat soft cheese called mascarpone — definitely not on the food list for lactose-intolerant people! Once again, silken soft tofu comes to the rescue as a substitute in this creamy confection.

SERVES 8

TIP

Separate eggs while cold, using three small bowls. Crack each egg over the first bowl, then separate the yolk into one side of the egg shell and the white into the other. Put the yolk in bowl two and the white in bowl three. This way, if you break one of the yolks while cracking the egg, you will not ruin all of the yolks and whites you have separated.

2	packages (each 10.25 oz/290 g) silken soft tofu	2
5	egg yolks	5
½ cup	granulated sugar	125 mL
½ cup	dark rum, divided	125 mL
3	egg whites	3
Pinch	salt	Pinch
½ cup	hot water	125 mL
1 tbsp	instant coffee granules	15 mL
1	package (7 oz/200 g) ladyfingers	1
¼ cup	unsweetened cocoa powder	50 mL

1. Using a sieve, drain tofu.

2. In a deep mixing bowl, using an electric mixer, beat egg yolks, sugar and ¼ cup (50 mL) of the rum for 3 to 4 minutes, or until thickened.

3. In a heavy saucepan, over medium heat, cook egg yolk mixture, whisking to prevent curdling, until thick enough to coat the back of a spoon, about 5 minutes. Do not boil. Let cool, then strain through a sieve.

4. Meanwhile, in a clean bowl, using clean beaters, beat egg whites and salt on high speed until stiff peaks form. Set aside.

Nutritional value
Per serving

Calories	267
Protein	9 g
Fat	7 g
Carbohydrate	32 g
Dietary Fiber	0 g
Calcium	51 mg

Percent of calories from

Protein	13%
Fat	24%
Carbohydrate	48%

5. In a food processor or blender, purée drained tofu. Add rum custard and combine. Remove to a clean bowl and fold in beaten egg white.

6. In a small bowl, mix hot water with instant coffee to dissolve; stir in remaining rum. Dip ladyfingers into coffee mixture and arrange some in the bottom of a glass bowl. Spread with about one-third of the rum custard; arrange ladyfingers in a single layer on top. Spread another third of custard on top of ladyfingers; top with remaining ladyfingers. Spread with remaining rum custard. Sift cocoa over entire dessert. Cover and refrigerate until ready to serve.

This recipe contains raw egg whites. If the food safety of raw eggs is a concern for you, use pasteurized eggs. Many grocery stores now carry pasteurized eggs in their shells.

MAKE AHEAD

Cover and store in the refrigerator for up to 1 day.

Fudge Pudding

Serve this hot and comforting self-saucing pudding with Vanilla Ice Cream (see recipe, page 236) or Yogurt Sauce (see recipe, page 256), if yogurt is tolerated.

MAKES 6 SERVINGS

TIP

This is an updated version of old-fashioned self-saucing chocolate pudding. The coffee, cocoa and cinnamon give the pudding a taste reminiscent of cappuccino.

● *Preheat oven to 350°F (180°C)*
● *6-cup (1.5 L) baking dish, greased*

1 cup	all-purpose flour	250 mL
1/2 cup	granulated sugar	125 mL
1/4 cup	unsweetened cocoa powder	50 mL
1 tsp	baking soda	5 mL
1 tsp	baking powder	5 mL
1/4 tsp	ground cinnamon	1 mL
1/4 tsp	salt	1 mL
1 1/2 tsp	instant coffee granules	7 mL
1/2 cup	hot water	125 mL
2 tbsp	vegetable oil	25 mL

Sauce

1/4 cup	packed brown sugar	50 mL
1/4 cup	unsweetened cocoa powder	50 mL
1/4 cup	currants, rinsed	50 mL
1 tbsp	dark rum (or 1 tsp/5 mL vanilla)	15 mL
1 tbsp	instant coffee granules	15 mL
1 1/2 cups	boiling water	375 mL

1. In a medium bowl, stir together flour, sugar, cocoa, baking soda, baking powder, cinnamon and salt.

2. Dissolve instant coffee in hot water (or use 1/2 cup/125 mL double-strength perked coffee); stir into dry mixture, along with oil. Spread in prepared baking dish.

Nutritional value
Per serving (with sauce)

Calories	250
Protein	4 g
Fat	6 g
Carbohydrate	49 g
Dietary Fiber	1 g
Calcium	37 mg

Percent of calories from

Protein	6%
Fat	18%
Carbohydrate	73%

3. *Prepare the sauce:* In a small mixing bowl, stir together brown sugar, cocoa, currants and rum. Dissolve instant coffee in boiling water (or use 1$\frac{1}{2}$ cups/375 mL double-strength perked coffee); gradually whisk into bowl. Pour over batter in dish.

4. Bake in preheated oven for 40 to 45 minutes, or until bubbly and pudding has risen to top.

Chocolate Mousse

Rich with cream and eggs, chocolate mousse is a classic finale to a special dinner. This recipe is lactose-free but has all the same rich flavor. Without the cream, it is lower in fat too!

TIP

Toasting nuts intensifies their flavor. To toast almonds, bake in preheated 350°F (180°C) oven for 10 to 12 minutes, or until golden brown and fragrant.

MAKE AHEAD

Cover and store in the refrigerator for up to 1 day.

¾ cup	granulated sugar	175 mL
½ cup	unsweetened cocoa powder	125 mL
¼ cup	water	50 mL
1 tbsp	instant coffee granules	15 mL
5	eggs, separated	5
¼ tsp	salt	1 mL
2 tbsp	orange-flavored liqueur (or 2 tbsp/25 mL fortified orange juice concentrate)	25 mL
¼ cup	toasted sliced almonds (see tip, at left)	50 mL

1. In a small saucepan, stir together sugar, cocoa, water and coffee granules; cook over medium heat, stirring frequently, for 3 to 4 minutes, or until smooth and thickened.

2. Beat egg yolks; whisk into cocoa mixture and cook for about 1 minute. Let cool.

3. Meanwhile, in a clean bowl, using an electric mixer, beat egg whites and salt on high speed until stiff peaks form.

4. Stir orange-flavored liqueur into cooled cocoa mixture. Fold in egg whites.

5. Spoon into glass dishes, demitasse cups or wine glasses. Sprinkle with toasted almonds.

> This recipe contains raw egg whites. If the food safety of raw eggs is a concern for you, use pasteurized eggs. Many grocery stores now carry pasteurized eggs in their shells.

Nutritional value
Per serving

Calories	225
Protein	7 g
Fat	8 g
Carbohydrate	33 g
Dietary Fiber	1 g
Calcium (a source)	63 mg

Percent of calories from

Protein	12%
Fat	30%
Carbohydrate	54%

Biscuit Tortoni

These dainty Italian confections are ideal for entertaining because they can be made ahead and kept frozen. Look for amaretti biscuits in Italian grocery stores.

MAKES 8 SERVINGS

TIP

Whenever you're working with eggs, especially if you're using raw egg whites in a dessert, check the expiry date on the carton. Discard any eggs with cracks. Always buy them refrigerated and keep them refrigerated. Wash hands thoroughly after separating eggs.

MAKE AHEAD

Store in the freezer for up to 2 days.

Nutritional value
Per serving

Calories	173
Protein	5 g
Fat	6 g
Carbohydrate	24 g
Dietary Fiber	1 g
Calcium	43 mg

Percent of calories from

Protein	12%
Fat	30%
Carbohydrate	54%

4	egg whites (or ½ cup/125 mL pasteurized liquid egg whites)	4
¼ cup	granulated sugar	50 mL
2 tbsp	amaretto liqueur (or 1 tsp/5 mL almond extract)	25 mL
1 cup	amaretti biscuits	250 mL
½ cup	coarsely chopped drained maraschino cherries (optional)	125 mL
½ cup	toasted chopped unblanched almonds (see tip, page 234)	125 mL
½ tsp	almond extract	2 mL

1. In a large bowl, using an electric mixer, beat egg whites on high speed until soft peaks form. Gradually beat in sugar, 1 tablespoonful (15 mL) at a time, until stiff peaks form. Fold in liqueur.

2. In a small bowl, using your hands, crush amaretti biscuits to make ½ cup (125 mL) coarse crumbs.

3. Fold half the crumbs, cherries (if using), almonds and almond extract into egg white mixture. Spoon into 8 large pretty muffin papers or dainty serving cups. Sprinkle with the remaining crumbs. Cover with plastic wrap and freeze for at least 4 hours.

> This recipe contains raw egg whites. If the food safety of raw eggs is a concern for you, use the pasteurized liquid egg whites instead.

Vanilla Ice Cream

The vanilla bean gives the ice cream an intense flavor and a distinctive speckled appearance.
Vanilla beans are available in gourmet shops, delicatessens and some bulk food stores.

MAKES ABOUT 4 CUPS (1 L) OR 8 SERVINGS

TIPS

To ensure a smooth product, strain egg yolk mixture through a sieve, using the back of a spoon to push it through, to remove any lumps caused from curdling.

If you don't have cream of tartar on hand, simply substitute a pinch of salt. Cream of tartar helps stabilize the egg white into firm peaks.

MAKE AHEAD

Store in the freezer for up to 2 days.

6	egg yolks	6
⅔ cup	granulated sugar, divided	150 mL
1	vanilla bean	1
½ cup	fortified soy milk or lactose-free milk	125 mL
4	egg whites	4
½ tsp	cream of tartar	2 mL

1. In a medium bowl, using an electric mixer, beat egg yolks and ⅓ cup (75 mL) of the sugar until thickened and lemony in color, about 2 minutes.

2. With a sharp knife, cut vanilla bean in half lengthwise; add to egg yolks, along with milk.

3. In a heavy stainless steel saucepan, cook yolk mixture, whisking, over medium-low heat for 5 to 8 minutes, or until thick enough to coat the back of a spoon. Do not boil. Immediately remove from heat; strain through a sieve into a bowl. Cover and let cool to room temperature.

4. In a clean bowl, using clean beaters, beat egg whites and cream of tartar on high speed until soft peaks form. Gradually beat in remaining sugar, 1 tablespoonful (15 mL) at a time, until stiff peaks form.

5. Fold about one-third of the egg white mixture into cooled custard. Fold in remaining egg whites.

6. Spoon mixture into a shallow pan; cover with plastic wrap and freeze for at least 4 hours.

Variations

Lemon Ice Cream: Substitute $1/2$ cup (125 mL) freshly squeezed lemon juice for the vanilla bean and milk in Step 2. Add 1 tbsp (15 mL) grated lemon zest after straining in Step 3.

Coffee Ice Cream: Substitute 2 tbsp (25 mL) instant coffee granules dissolved in 2 tbsp (25 mL) water for the vanilla bean and milk in Step 2. Add 1 tsp (5 mL) vanilla in Step 5.

Mocha Ice Cream: Substitute 1 cup (250 mL) fortified soy milk or lactose-free milk, $1/2$ cup (125 mL) unsweetened cocoa powder and 2 tbsp (25 mL) instant coffee granules for the vanilla bean and milk in Step 2; beat until dissolved. Add 1 tsp (5 mL) vanilla in Step 5.

Strawberry Ice Cream: Purée 2 cups (500 mL) fresh or frozen strawberries and substitute for vanilla bean and milk in Step 2.

Mango Sorbet

Be sure to use fully ripe mangoes. Mangoes are ripe when they have a distinct sweet fragrance and a deep orange color and feel tender to the touch.

MAKES ABOUT 2 CUPS (500 ML) OR 4 SERVINGS

MAKE AHEAD

Store in the freezer for up to 2 days.

● *Ice cream maker (optional)*

3	large mangoes	3
½ cup	water	125 mL
½ cup	granulated sugar	125 mL
¼ cup	freshly squeezed lime juice	50 mL

1. Scrape mango flesh away from pit and skin. In a food processor, using pulsing action, purée flesh until smooth (or mash with a fork until smooth), to make about 1½ cups (375 mL).

2. In a small saucepan, bring water and sugar to a boil over high heat; reduce heat to medium-low and simmer for 2 minutes, until heated through and slightly thickened. Let cool to room temperature.

3. Stir lime juice and cooled syrup into mango purée until well combined.

4. Freeze in ice cream maker according to manufacturer's directions or in a shallow pan covered with plastic wrap for at least 4 hours.

Nutritional value
Per serving (½ cup/125 mL)

Calories	201
Protein	1 g
Fat	0 g
Carbohydrate	53 g
Dietary Fiber (a high source)	4 g
Calcium	18 mg

Percent of calories from

Protein	2%
Fat	2%
Carbohydrate	97%

Banana Sorbet

For best flavor and sweetness, use overripe bananas. This sorbet is so creamy, it's more like ice cream.

TIP

To speed the cooling of the sugar syrup, pour into a shallow container and refrigerate for 40 to 45 minutes.

MAKE AHEAD

Store in the freezer for up to 2 days.

● *Ice cream maker (optional)*

3	large bananas	3
1/4 cup	freshly squeezed lemon juice	50 mL
1 cup	water	250 mL
1 cup	granulated sugar	250 mL

1. In a food processor, using pulsing action, purée banana until smooth (or mash with a fork until smooth), to make about 1 1/2 cups (375 mL). Add lemon juice and stir or purée to combine.

2. In a small saucepan, bring water and sugar to a boil over high heat; reduce heat to medium and simmer for 2 minutes, until slightly thickened. Let cool to room temperature.

3. Stir cooled syrup into banana purée.

4. Freeze in ice cream maker according to manufacturer's directions or in a shallow pan covered with plastic wrap for at least 4 hours.

If you have ripe bananas and aren't ready to use them, pop them into the freezer with the skins on until you're ready to transform them into sorbet or some other treat. Peel while still frozen and defrost for a few minutes before mashing.

Nutritional value
Per serving (1/2 cup/125 mL)

Calories	138
Protein	1 g
Fat	0 g
Carbohydrate	36 g
Dietary Fiber	1 g
Calcium	4 mg

Percent of calories from

Protein	1%
Fat	1%
Carbohydrate	97%

Apricot Sorbet

For a sophisticated finale, drizzle a spoonful of apricot brandy or orange liqueur over each serving.

MAKES ABOUT 2 CUPS (500 ML) OR 4 SERVINGS

MAKE AHEAD

Store in the freezer for up to 2 days.

● Ice cream maker (optional)

1 cup	dried apricots	250 mL
2 cups	water, divided	500 mL
1 cup	granulated sugar	250 mL
¼ cup	freshly squeezed lemon juice	50 mL

1. In a small saucepan, cover apricots with 1 cup (250 mL) of the water; bring to a boil over high heat. Reduce heat to medium and simmer until very tender and water has been absorbed, about 5 minutes.

2. Meanwhile, in another saucepan, bring the remaining water and sugar to a boil over high heat; reduce heat to medium and simmer for 2 minutes, until slightly thickened. Let cool to room temperature.

3. In a food processor, using pulsing action, purée apricots, lemon juice and sugar syrup until smooth. (If little bits of fruit remain, they will add texture to the sorbet.)

4. Freeze in ice cream maker according to manufacturer's directions or in a shallow pan covered with plastic wrap for at least 4 hours.

Nutritional value
Per serving (½ cup/125 mL)

Calories	290
Protein	2 g
Fat	0 g
Carbohydrate	76 g
Dietary Fiber	1 g
Calcium	22 mg

Percent of calories from

Protein	2%
Fat	1%
Carbohydrate	98%

Sauces, Spreads and Toppings

These lactose-free sauces, spreads and toppings provide delicious alternatives for those with lactose intolerance so they need not feel deprived. The trick is to find suitable substitutes. Tofu, lactose-free milk and soy milk replace the usual cream, milk and sour cream so frequently required in classic cream-based sauces. Herbs and seasonings jazz up sauces for pasta and meat, and flavored crumb mixtures replace large quantities of cheese.

Basic Cream Sauce 242

Basic Béchamel Sauce for
   Chicken Dishes. 243

Pesto Sauce 244

Green Sauce. 245

Dill Mustard Sauce. 246

Tofu Cream. 247

Tofu "Sour Cream" for
   Baked Potatoes 248

Gremolata Bread Crumbs 249

Rosemary Sun-Dried Tomato
   Crumb Topping. 250

Whole Wheat Croutons. 251

Pumpkin Butter 252

Pear Butter. 253

Apple Butter 254

Lemon Butter 255

Yogurt Sauce 256

Amaretto Cream 257

Vanilla Cream Filling 258

Quick Strawberry Sauce 259

Cappuccino Sauce 260

Old-Fashioned Chocolate Sauce 261

Basic Custard Sauce. 262

Basic Cream Sauce

A basic cream sauce, also called a béchamel sauce, is considered a "mother" sauce, that is, the foundation for numerous other sauces, used in countless casseroles and dishes.

MAKES ABOUT 1 CUP (250 ML)

TIPS

Heating the milk in the microwave, in a microwave-safe measuring cup, speeds up the cooking process.

If you're using soy milk, you may have to add extra seasoning, as soy milk has a flat taste. A sprinkling of chopped fresh parsley will improve the tan color.

2 tbsp	all-purpose flour	25 mL
2 tbsp	vegetable oil	25 mL
1 cup	lactose-free milk or fortified soy milk, heated to steaming	250 mL
1	bay leaf	1
1/2 tsp	salt	2 mL
Pinch	freshly ground black pepper	Pinch
Pinch	ground nutmeg	Pinch

1. In a heavy saucepan, over medium-high heat, stir together flour and oil until smooth. Cook until pale brown, about 2 minutes. Remove from heat.

2. Gradually whisk in hot milk. Return to heat and add bay leaf, salt, pepper and nutmeg. Cook, whisking, until thickened, about 2 minutes. Remove from heat and discard bay leaf.

Variations

Cheese Sauce: If tolerated, stir in 2 tbsp to 1/3 cup (25 to 75 mL) shredded old Cheddar or freshly grated Parmesan cheese to the finished sauce.

Add 2 tbsp (25 mL) chopped fresh parsley or herbs of your choice.

Nutritional value
Per serving (2 tbsp/25 mL)

Calories	51
Protein	1 g
Fat	4 g
Carbohydrate	3 g
Dietary Fiber	0 g
Calcium	40 mg

Percent of calories from

Protein	10%
Fat	66%
Carbohydrate	25%

Basic Béchamel Sauce
for Chicken Dishes

This lactose-free version of béchamel sauce has a velvety texture and rich flavor — the perfect complement to any chicken casserole calling for a cream or béchamel sauce.

MAKES ABOUT 2 CUPS (500 ML)

MAKE AHEAD

Spoon into an airtight container and store in the refrigerator for up to 1 day.

3 tbsp	all-purpose flour	45 mL
2 tbsp	vegetable oil or chicken fat	25 mL
1	bay leaf	1
1 cup	chicken stock	250 mL
¼ cup	white wine or sherry	50 mL
1 cup	lactose-free milk or fortified soy milk	250 mL
	Salt and freshly ground black pepper	

1. In a medium saucepan, stir together flour and oil until smooth. Heat over medium-high heat until bubbly, about 2 minutes. Remove from heat.

2. Add bay leaf and gradually whisk in chicken stock. Return to medium heat and cook, stirring, for 4 to 5 minutes, or until thickened and smooth. Stir in wine; cook for 1 minute. Gradually whisk in milk; increase heat to medium-high and cook, stirring, until thickened, about 5 minutes. Discard bay leaf. Season to taste with salt and pepper.

Variation

Mushroom Cream Sauce: Cook 1½ cups (375 mL) sliced mushrooms in vegetable oil over medium-high heat until liquid is released, about 5 minutes. Sprinkle with 3 tbsp (45 mL) flour and stir until smooth. Continue with Step 2 of recipe.

Nutritional value
Per serving (½ cup/125 mL)

Calories	132
Protein	4 g
Fat	8 g
Carbohydrate	8 g
Dietary Fiber	0 g
Calcium	80 mg

Percent of calories from

Protein	12%
Fat	57%
Carbohydrate	24%

Pesto Sauce

Pesto is an Italian green sauce made with basil, olive oil, Parmesan cheese and pine nuts. When you have a jar of pesto in the refrigerator or freezer (yes, it freezes like a dream!) you have a culinary insurance policy tucked into your apron pocket. It is invaluable as a tossing sauce for pasta, as a base for vinaigrette, as a spread on fish or chicken, as a sandwich spread, as a base for dip… the list goes on.

MAKES ABOUT 1⅓ CUPS (325 ML)

MAKE AHEAD

Spoon pesto into an airtight container and store in the refrigerator for up to 2 weeks. Or freeze measured amounts in an ice cube tray, then place cubes in a freezer bag and store in the freezer for up to 2 months.

Nutritional value
Per serving (1½ tbsp/22 mL)

Calories	226
Protein	3 g
Fat	24 g
Carbohydrate	2 g
Dietary Fiber	1 g
Calcium (a source)	63 mg

Percent of calories from

Protein	5%
Fat	92%
Carbohydrate	3%

- *Preheat oven to 350°F (180°C)*
- *Baking sheet*

¼ cup	pine nuts	50 mL
2 cups	packed fresh basil leaves	500 mL
¼ cup	freshly grated Parmesan cheese (optional, if tolerated)	50 mL
3	cloves garlic, minced	3
½ tsp	salt	2 mL
¼ tsp	freshly ground black pepper	1 mL
¾ cup	extra-virgin olive oil	175 mL

1. Spread pine nuts on baking sheet. Toast in preheated oven until golden and fragrant, about 10 minutes. Let cool.

2. In a food processor, using pulsing action, chop pine nuts, basil, cheese (if using), garlic, salt and pepper until finely chopped. With motor running, gradually add oil through feed tube and process until pesto is emulsified.

Variation

For a winter version of this recipe, substitute an equal amount of fresh parsley for the fresh basil and add 2 tbsp (25 mL) dried basil.

Green Sauce

This is my favorite all-purpose sauce to serve with any fish, especially salmon. It works well as a dip for vegetables too!

MAKES 1 CUP (250 ML)

MAKE AHEAD

Spoon into an airtight container and store in the refrigerator for up to 3 days.

1	package (10.25 oz/290 g) silken soft tofu	1
¼ cup	chopped fresh dill	50 mL
¼ cup	chopped fresh parsley	50 mL
¼ cup	chopped green onions	50 mL
2 tbsp	freshly squeezed lemon juice	25 mL
2 tbsp	light mayonnaise	25 mL
½ tsp	salt	2 mL
¼ tsp	freshly ground black pepper	1 mL

1. Using a sieve, drain tofu.

2. In a food processor, purée drained tofu, dill, parsley, onions, lemon juice, mayonnaise, salt and pepper.

Nutritional value
Per serving (2 tbsp/25 mL)

Calories	41
Protein	2 g
Fat	3 g
Carbohydrate	2 g
Dietary Fiber	0 g
Calcium	24 mg

Percent of calories from

Protein	18%
Fat	61%
Carbohydrate	21%

Dill Mustard Sauce

Serve this with anything salmon — Salmon Loaf (see recipe, page 154), Easy Salmon Pie (see recipe, page 150) or simply a salmon sandwich. It adds zing! In fact, it is good with chicken and ham too.

MAKES ABOUT 1½ CUPS (375 ML)

TIP

Do not be intimidated by how big a bunch of dill is. It reduces to very little once the stems are removed.

MAKE AHEAD

Spoon into an airtight container and store in the refrigerator for up to 3 weeks.

1	bunch fresh dill, stems removed	1
¼ cup	granulated sugar	50 mL
½ cup	vegetable oil	125 mL
½ cup	Dijon mustard	125 mL
¼ cup	red wine vinegar	50 mL

1. In a food processor, using pulsing action, chop dill and sugar until dill is finely chopped. With motor running, add vegetable oil, mustard and vinegar through the feed tube and process until smooth.

Nutritional value
Per serving (2 tbsp/25 mL)

Calories	72
Protein	0 g
Fat	7 g
Carbohydrate	3 g
Dietary Fiber	0 g
Calcium	1 mg

Percent of calories from

Protein	0%
Fat	83%
Carbohydrate	17%

Tofu Cream

Tofu makes a lower-fat, calcium-enriched, mayonnaise-like dressing. It works well as a spread or as a base for other creamy dressings such as ranch and Thousand Island.

MAKES ABOUT 1 CUP (250 ML)

MAKE AHEAD

Spoon into an airtight container and store in the refrigerator for up to 2 days.

1	package (10.25 oz/290 g) silken soft tofu	1
2 tbsp	freshly squeezed lemon juice	25 mL
1 tbsp	vegetable oil	15 mL
2 tsp	Dijon mustard	10 mL
1 tsp	salt	5 mL
1 tsp	granulated sugar	5 mL
1/4 tsp	freshly ground black pepper	1 mL
Pinch	cayenne pepper	Pinch

1. Using a sieve, drain tofu.
2. In a food processor, using pulsing action, purée drained tofu, lemon juice, oil, mustard, salt, sugar, pepper and cayenne.

Nutritional value
Per serving (1 tbsp/15 mL)

Calories	20
Protein	1 g
Fat	1 g
Carbohydrate	1 g
Dietary Fiber	0 g
Calcium	7 mg

Percent of calories from

Protein	18%
Fat	64%
Carbohydrate	18%

Tofu "Sour Cream" for Baked Potatoes

You don't need to feel deprived when you serve this tofu cream on your baked potatoes or with any food, such as tortilla chips and crudités, with which you would normally want some sour cream.

MAKES ABOUT 1¼ CUPS (300 ML)

MAKE AHEAD

Spoon into an airtight container and store in the refrigerator for up to 2 days.

1	package (10.25 oz/290 g) silken firm tofu	1
1 tbsp	freshly squeezed lemon juice	15 mL
1 tbsp	vegetable oil	15 mL
½ tsp	salt	2 mL
½ tsp	granulated sugar	2 mL

Zesty Toppers (optional)

¼ cup	chopped red bell pepper	50 mL
¼ cup	chopped jalapeño pepper	50 mL
2 tbsp	chopped black olives	25 mL

1. Using a sieve, drain tofu.

2. In a food processor, purée drained tofu, lemon juice, oil, salt and sugar.

3. *Add the Zesty Toppers (if using):* For added zest, stir in red pepper, jalapeño pepper and olives.

Plain Tofu Cream

Nutritional value
Per serving (2 tbsp/25 mL)

Calories	26
Protein	2 g
Fat	2 g
Carbohydrate	1 g
Dietary Fiber	0 g
Calcium	8 mg

Percent of calories from

Protein	25%
Fat	62%
Carbohydrate	13%

Gremolata Bread Crumbs

The Mediterranean flavors combine in this zesty mixture that's ideal as a coating or stuffing for fish, seafood, poultry, or veal or as a topping for pasta.

MAKES ABOUT 2½ CUPS (625 ML)

MAKE AHEAD

Place in an airtight container and store in the refrigerator for up to 2 days or in the freezer for up to 2 months.

2 cups	fresh bread crumbs from Italian or French bread	500 mL
½ cup	chopped fresh parsley	125 mL
2 tbsp	grated lemon zest	25 mL
1 tbsp	freshly grated Parmesan cheese (optional, if tolerated)	15 mL
1 tbsp	extra-virgin olive oil	15 mL
1 tsp	dried tarragon	5 mL
½ tsp	salt	2 mL
½ tsp	dried basil	2 mL
¼ tsp	freshly ground black pepper	1 mL

1. In a medium bowl, combine bread crumbs, parsley, lemon zest, cheese (if using), oil, tarragon, salt, basil and pepper. Taste and adjust seasonings.

Seasoned bread crumbs are a great flavor substitute in many recipes where cheese or cream sauces play a major role. Commercial bread crumb coatings may contain lactose in the form of milk solids. Making your own bread crumbs without lactose is easy. Simply break up a piece of bread and process in the blender or food processor. For variety, use whole wheat, rye or mixed-grain breads.

Nutritional value
Per serving (½ cup/125 mL)

Calories	191
Protein	6 g
Fat	5 g
Carbohydrate	30 g
Dietary Fiber (a source)	2 g
Calcium (a source)	86 mg

Percent of calories from

Protein	12%
Fat	24%
Carbohydrate	63%

Rosemary Sun-Dried Tomato Crumb Topping

Use this robust-flavored crumb topping for pasta dishes such as lasagna, or as a coating or stuffing for meat or poultry.

MAKES ABOUT 1⅓ CUPS (325 ML)

1 cup	fresh bread crumbs (from Italian or French bread)	250 mL
¼ cup	chopped fresh parsley	50 mL
2 tbsp	diced sun-dried tomato, packed in oil	25 mL
1 tbsp	freshly grated Parmesan cheese (optional, if tolerated)	15 mL
1 tbsp	extra-virgin olive oil	15 mL
½ tsp	dried basil	2 mL
Pinch	dried rosemary	Pinch
Pinch	freshly ground black pepper	Pinch

1. In a medium bowl, combine bread crumbs, parsley, tomato, cheese (if using), olive oil, basil, rosemary and pepper. Taste and adjust seasonings.

MAKE AHEAD

Place in an airtight container and store in the refrigerator for up to 2 days or in the freezer for up to 2 months.

Sun-dried tomatoes can be purchased dried in a package or in oil in a jar. The oil-packed ones are more expensive. To reconstitute dry-packed tomatoes, place in a saucepan and cover with hot water; add a bay leaf and bring to a boil. Reduce heat and simmer for 5 to 10 minutes, or until tomatoes are tender; drain. May be used at this point, but for more flavor, place in a jar and cover with extra-virgin olive oil and crushed garlic (and basil or fennel seeds, if you wish). Refrigerate for up to 2 weeks.

Nutritional value
Per serving (⅓ cup/75 mL)

Calories	147
Protein	5 g
Fat	6 g
Carbohydrate	21 g
Dietary Fiber (a source)	2 g
Calcium (a source)	80 mg

Percent of calories from

Protein	12%
Fat	33%
Carbohydrate	55%

Whole Wheat Croutons

Commercial croutons can be a hidden source of lactose — either in the bread or seasoning. Check the label for skim milk powder or milk solids. Better yet, make your own to be on the safe side, such as these "too good to be true" croutons. Beware: they taste so good for nibbling, there may not be any left for the soup.

MAKES ABOUT 1⅔ CUPS (400 ML)

- Preheat oven to 375°F (190°C)
- Baking sheets

2 tbsp	extra-virgin olive oil	25 mL
1	clove garlic, minced	1
4	slices day-old whole wheat bread	4

1. In a small bowl, combine oil and garlic. Using a pastry brush, paint lightly over both sides of bread.

2. Trim crusts and cut bread into ½-inch (1 cm) cubes. Place on baking sheets and bake in preheated oven for 20 to 25 minutes, or until golden brown.

Nutritional value
Per serving (⅓ cup/75 mL)

Calories	96
Protein	2 g
Fat	5 g
Carbohydrate	11 g
Dietary Fiber	1 g
Calcium	20 mg

Percent of calories from

Protein	8%
Fat	46%
Carbohydrate	45%

Pumpkin Butter

This is a wonderful spread for pumpkin muffins or seed and nut bread.

TIP

When a recipe specifies stainless steel saucepans, it's because the metal will not react with the acid of the ingredients. A glass saucepan would work just as well.

MAKE AHEAD

Spoon into an airtight container and store in the refrigerator for up to 5 days.

2 cups	pumpkin purée (not pie filling)	500 mL
1/2 cup	apple juice	125 mL
1/4 cup	fancy molasses	50 mL
1 tbsp	packed brown sugar	15 mL
1/2 tsp	ground cinnamon	2 mL
1/4 tsp	ground cloves	1 mL
1/4 tsp	ground ginger	1 mL
Pinch	salt	Pinch

1. In a large stainless steel saucepan, combine pumpkin purée, apple juice, molasses, brown sugar, cinnamon, cloves, ginger and salt. Bring to a boil over high heat; reduce heat to medium and simmer, uncovered, until thickened, about 5 minutes. Let cool.

Nutritional value
Per serving (2 tbsp/25 mL)

Calories	28
Protein	0 g
Fat	0 g
Carbohydrate	7 g
Dietary Fiber	1 g
Calcium	44 mg

Percent of calories from

Protein	5%
Fat	3%
Carbohydrate	92%

Pear Butter

Pear butter is a delectable, thick, spiced spread for pancakes, toast and muffins or condiment with pork or poultry. It's so yummy, you just might eat it by the spoonful too!

MAKES ABOUT 2 CUPS (500 ML)

TIP

You won't need butter when you have these flavorful spreads. Be sure to make pear butter in the autumn when pears are cheap and plentiful. Each pear variety will give a different flavor and texture to the spread.

MAKE AHEAD

Spoon into an airtight container and store in the refrigerator for up to 1 week or in the freezer for up to 3 months.

4	pears, peeled, cored and diced	4
1 cup	water	250 mL
½ cup	liquid honey	125 mL
1	strip lemon peel	1
2 tbsp	freshly squeezed lemon juice	25 mL
1	cinnamon stick	1

1. In a large stainless steel saucepan, combine pears, water, honey, lemon peel, lemon juice and cinnamon stick. Bring to a boil over high heat; reduce heat to medium and simmer, stirring, until pears are very tender, about 15 minutes.

2. Discard peel and cinnamon stick. Purée in a food processor or beat with a fork until smooth.

Nutritional value
Per serving (2 tbsp/25 mL)

Calories	43
Protein	0 g
Fat	0 g
Carbohydrate	11 g
Dietary Fiber	0 g
Calcium	3 mg

Percent of calories from

Protein	1%
Fat	0%
Carbohydrate	99%

Apple Butter

An old-fashioned recipe, this spicy spread is the perfect companion to pancakes or pork.

MAKES ABOUT 2 CUPS (500 ML)

4 cups	apples, peeled, cored and chopped (about 6 medium)	1 L
2 cups	unsweetened apple juice	500 mL
1/3 cup	liquid honey	75 mL
1/2 tsp	ground cinnamon	2 mL
1/4 tsp	ground cloves	1 mL

MAKE AHEAD

Spoon into an airtight container and store in the refrigerator for up to 1 week.

1. In a large stainless steel saucepan, combine apples, apple juice, honey, cinnamon and cloves. Bring to a boil over high heat; reduce heat to medium and simmer, uncovered, for 20 to 25 minutes, or until apples are soft and mushy.

2. For a super-smooth texture, purée in a blender or beat with a fork. Serve hot or cold.

Nutritional value
Per serving (2 tbsp/25 mL)

Calories	57
Protein	0 g
Fat	0 g
Carbohydrate	15 g
Dietary Fiber	0 g
Calcium	6 mg

Percent of calories from

Protein	1%
Fat	3%
Carbohydrate	96%

Lemon Butter

This classic, rich, creamy and intensely flavored spread is ideal for tea breads and jelly-roll slices and as a filling for tarts and meringues.

MAKES ABOUT 1 CUP (250 ML)

MAKE AHEAD

Spoon into an airtight container and store in the refrigerator for up to 1 week or in the freezer for up to 1 month.

2	eggs	2
1 cup	granulated sugar	250 mL
1 tbsp	grated lemon zest	15 mL
½ cup	freshly squeezed lemon juice	125 mL

1. In a medium bowl, whisk together eggs, sugar, lemon zest and lemon juice until smooth.

2. Pour into a medium stainless steel saucepan and cook, whisking, over medium heat until just bubbling, thickened and smooth, about 10 minutes. Let cool.

Variations

Lime Butter: Substitute lime zest and juice for lemon zest and juice.

Citrus Butter: Use a combination of lemon, lime and orange to make up the amounts of zest and juice in the recipe.

Nutritional value
Per serving (1 tbsp/15 mL)

Calories	110
Protein	1 g
Fat	1 g
Carbohydrate	26 g
Dietary Fiber	0 g
Calcium	6 mg

Percent of calories from

Protein	2%
Fat	6%
Carbohydrate	92%

Yogurt Sauce

No one will ever guess the simplicity and healthy base of this delicious creamy sauce. If time is tight, simply stir the brown sugar and flavoring into the undrained yogurt for an instant sauce. It can be served with fresh berries, over puddings or as a sauce for cakes.

MAKES 1 CUP (250 ML)

MAKE AHEAD

Spoon into an airtight container and store in the refrigerator for up to 1 day.

2 cups	plain yogurt (see tip, below)	500 mL
1/4 cup	packed brown sugar	50 mL
1 tbsp	dark rum, amaretto liqueur or vanilla	15 mL

1. Spoon yogurt into a sieve lined with two layers of cheesecloth, or into a coffee filter over a bowl. Cover and refrigerate for about 4 hours, until reduced by about half, or overnight.

2. In a small bowl, stir together reduced yogurt, sugar and rum until well combined.

Many people with lactose intolerance find that they can digest yogurt with natural bacteria. The bacteria help break down the lactose. If you can digest yogurt, try to incorporate it into your diet as a calcium source. If regular yogurt is a problem for you, try the lactose-free yogurts now available in grocery stores.

Nutritional value
Per serving (1 tbsp/15 mL)

Calories	29
Protein	2 g
Fat	0 g
Carbohydrate	5 g
Dietary Fiber	0 g
Calcium	54 mg

Percent of calories from

Protein	21%
Fat	1%
Carbohydrate	69%

Amaretto Cream

Use this cream as a dip for fruit or as a sauce for desserts to replace whipping cream.

MAKES ABOUT 1⅓ CUPS (325 ML)

MAKE AHEAD

Cover and store in the refrigerator for up to 4 hours.

1	package (10.25 oz/290 g) silken soft tofu	1
¼ cup	granulated sugar	50 mL
3 tbsp	amaretto liqueur	45 mL
½ tsp	grated lemon zest	2 mL

1. Using a sieve, drain tofu.
2. In a food processor, purée drained tofu, sugar, amaretto and lemon zest. Pour into a serving bowl.

Nutritional value
Per serving (2 tbsp/25 mL)

Calories	49
Protein	1 g
Fat	1 g
Carbohydrate	8 g
Dietary Fiber	0 g
Calcium	8 mg

Percent of calories from

Protein	11%
Fat	15%
Carbohydrate	59%

Vanilla Cream Filling

This cream and its flavorful variations can be used for dessert toppings, cake toppings or tart fillings. Try them with pancakes or crêpes.

MAKES ABOUT 1 CUP (250 ML)

MAKE AHEAD

Spoon into an airtight container and store in the refrigerator for up to 2 days or in the freezer for up to 1 month. Stir before using.

1/3 cup	granulated sugar	75 mL
2 tbsp	cornstarch	25 mL
1/4 tsp	salt	1 mL
1	egg	1
1 cup	lactose-free milk	250 mL
1 tsp	vanilla	5 mL

1. In a small saucepan, whisk together sugar, cornstarch and salt. Gradually whisk in egg, milk and vanilla. Cook over medium heat, whisking frequently, until smooth and thickened, about 5 minutes. Remove from heat and cover surface directly with plastic wrap. Let cool.

Variations

Coffee Cream Filling: Stir 2 tsp (10 mL) instant coffee granules into 1 cup (250 mL) hot water; use instead of lactose-free milk.

Chocolate Cream Filling: Add 3 tbsp (50 mL) unsweetened cocoa powder to dry ingredients. Substitute fortified soy milk for lactose-free milk, if desired.

Mocha Cream Filling: Add 1 tbsp (15 mL) unsweetened cocoa powder to dry ingredients. Dissolve 1 tbsp (15 mL) instant coffee granules in 1 cup (250 mL) water or lactose-free milk; use instead of lactose-free milk.

Nutritional value
Per serving (2 tbsp/25 mL)

Calories	63
Protein	2 g
Fat	1 g
Carbohydrate	11 g
Dietary Fiber	0 g
Calcium	42 mg

Percent of calories from

Protein	11%
Fat	19%
Carbohydrate	71%

Quick Strawberry Sauce

This instant sauce always brings back happy memories of picking berries under a sunny sky — one of my favorite pastimes! It is perfect as a topping for ice creams, Orange Pancakes (see recipe, page 61), Yeast Blini (see recipe, page 63) or Currant Scones (see recipe, page 199).

MAKES ABOUT 2 CUPS (500 ML)

TIP

Frozen berries work equally well in this recipe.

MAKE AHEAD

Spoon into an airtight container and store in the refrigerator for up to 2 weeks.

4 cups	whole strawberries	1 L
1 cup	granulated sugar	250 mL
2 tbsp	cornstarch	25 mL
1 tsp	grated orange zest (optional)	5 mL

1. In a large saucepan, stir together strawberries, sugar, cornstarch and orange zest (if using). Bring to a boil over high heat; reduce heat to medium-low and simmer, stirring, until thickened, about 5 minutes. Let cool. (Mixture will thicken more after cooling.)

Variation

Quick Blueberry Sauce: Substitute blueberries for strawberries and lemon zest for orange zest.

Nutritional value
Per serving (2 tbsp/25 mL)

Calories	63
Protein	0 g
Fat	0 g
Carbohydrate	16 g
Dietary Fiber	1 g
Calcium	5 mg

Percent of calories from

Protein	1%
Fat	2%
Carbohydrate	97%

Cappuccino Sauce

Keep a jar of this versatile sauce in your refrigerator to serve over ices, drizzle over cake, use as a dip for fresh fruit or stir into soy milk or lactose-free milk for hot cocoa.

MAKES ABOUT 1⅓ CUPS (325 ML)

MAKE AHEAD

Spoon into an airtight container and store in the refrigerator for up to 2 weeks.

¾ cup	unsweetened cocoa powder	175 mL
¾ cup	granulated sugar	175 mL
1 tbsp	instant coffee granules	15 mL
1	cinnamon stick	1
1 tsp	vanilla	5 mL
Pinch	salt	Pinch
1 cup	hot water	250 mL

1. In a small saucepan, stir together cocoa, sugar, coffee granules, cinnamon stick, vanilla and salt. Place over medium heat and gradually whisk in hot water until smooth. Cook, stirring, until thickened, about 5 minutes. Discard cinnamon stick. Let cool.

Nutritional value
Per serving (2 tbsp/25 mL)

Calories	73
Protein	1 g
Fat	1 g
Carbohydrate	19 g
Dietary Fiber	0 g
Calcium	12 mg

Percent of calories from

Protein	6%
Fat	6%
Carbohydrate	87%

Old-Fashioned Chocolate Sauce

For those with lactose intolerance, combining Chocolate Sauce with hot lactose-free milk makes a delicious calcium-rich drink. If you are just getting used to the taste of fortified soy milk, try mixing it with this chocolate sauce. Remember that, although soy milk is nutritious, it is not a calcium source like cow's milk.

MAKES ABOUT ⅔ CUP (150 ML)

MAKE AHEAD

Spoon into an airtight container and store in the refrigerator for up to 2 weeks.

½ cup	unsweetened cocoa powder	125 mL
½ cup	granulated sugar	125 mL
½ cup	hot water	125 mL
2 tsp	instant coffee granules	10 mL
1 tsp	vanilla	5 mL

1. In a small saucepan, whisk together cocoa and sugar. Gradually whisk in water, coffee and vanilla until smooth. Cook over medium heat, stirring often, until glossy and thickened, about 5 minutes.

To make hot cocoa: In a small saucepan, stir 2 tsp (10 mL) chocolate sauce into 1 cup (250 mL) lactose-free milk. Cook over medium heat, stirring frequently, just until it starts to bubble, about 4 minutes. Pour into mug and serve.

Nutritional value
Per serving (2 tbsp/25 mL)

Calories	41
Protein	1 g
Fat	0 g
Carbohydrate	11 g
Dietary Fiber	0 g
Calcium	6 mg

Percent of calories from

Protein	6%
Fat	6%
Carbohydrate	88%

Basic Custard Sauce

Custard sauce is a classic dessert sauce. This rendition is easily digested by the lactose intolerant.

MAKES ABOUT 1 CUP (250 ML)

TIP

Once egg yolk is added to the milk mixture, whisk frequently to prevent curdling.

¾ cup	hot lactose-free milk or fortified soy milk	175 mL
1 tbsp	cornstarch	15 mL
1	egg yolk	1
2 tbsp	granulated sugar	25 mL
1 tsp	vanilla	5 mL

1. In a small saucepan, whisk together hot milk and cornstarch until smooth. Cook over medium heat, whisking often, until sauce thickens, about 1 minute.

2. Meanwhile, in a measuring cup, whisk together egg yolk, sugar and vanilla. Whisk a little of the milk mixture into the egg mixture, then pour into the milk mixture and whisk. Cook, whisking, until sauce is thick enough to coat the back of a spoon, about 2 minutes. Let cool.

Variation

Add 1 tsp (5 mL) grated lemon or orange zest to the egg yolk.

Nutritional value
Per serving (2 tbsp/25 mL)

Calories	34
Protein	1 g
Fat	1 g
Carbohydrate	5 g
Dietary Fiber	0 g
Calcium	31 mg

Percent of calories from

Protein	13%
Fat	23%
Carbohydrate	60%

Smoothies and Other Beverages

These luscious beverages are no longer taboo for the lactose intolerant. Fruit purées, juices, tofu, lactose-free milk and soy milk replace the usual milk in these thirst quenchers. Drink up!

Basic Berry Smoothie. 264

Tofu Fruit Smoothie 265

Yogurt Fruit Smoothie 266

Tropical Smoothies. 267

Banana Peanut Butter Smoothie . . . 268

Cappuccino 269

Café au Lait 270

Chocolate Milkshake 271

Basic Berry Smoothie

Fresh fruit smoothies make a great snack or a partial mini breakfast.

TIPS

You need at least three food groups at breakfast. Serve the smoothie with yogurt, if tolerated, or some almonds.

Ripe bananas are sweeter than less ripe bananas.

Choose orange juice fortified with calcium for a calcium boost.

1	banana, chopped	1
1 cup	fresh strawberries, blueberries or raspberries	250 mL
½ cup	fortified orange juice	125 mL

1. In a blender, purée banana, berries and orange juice. Pour into a glass and serve.

Nutritional value
Per serving

Calories	203
Protein	3 g
Fat	1 g
Carbohydrate	51 g
Dietary Fiber (a very high source)	6 g
Calcium (a high source)	176 mg

Percent of calories from

Protein	5%
Fat	4%
Carbohydrate	91%

Tofu Fruit Smoothie

This mini meal in a glass replaces the old-fashioned eggnog and provides calcium if you use tofu made with calcium sulfate or calcium chloride. Make it with your kids' favorite fruit and serve with a colorful straw. It's sure to be a hit.

MAKES 2 SERVINGS

1	package (10.25 oz/290 g) silken soft tofu	1
1	banana	1
1 cup	fruit juice (orange, apple or cranberry)	250 mL
1 cup	berries, such as strawberries or blueberries (optional)	250 mL

1. In blender or food processor, purée tofu, banana, fruit juice and berries (if using) until smooth. Pour into glasses and serve immediately.

Nutritional value
Per serving

Calories	215
Protein	8 g
Fat	5 g
Carbohydrate	38 g
Dietary Fiber (a source)	3 g
Calcium (a source)	63 mg

Percent of calories from

Protein	14%
Fat	19%
Carbohydrate	67%

Yogurt Fruit Smoothie

If yogurt is tolerated, a yogurt fruit smoothie is a great way to get both calcium and some of your daily servings of fruit.

MAKES 2 SERVINGS

1 cup	very ripe fruit (such as mango, banana or orange), chopped	250 mL
¾ cup	fruit-flavored yogurt	175 g
½ cup	fortified orange juice	125 mL

1. In a blender, purée fruit, yogurt and orange juice. Pour into glasses and serve.

Variation

Try this with applesauce and apple juice.

Nutritional value
Per serving

Calories	201
Protein	6 g
Fat	1 g
Carbohydrate	46 g
Dietary Fiber (a source)	2 g
Calcium (a high source)	257 mg

Percent of calories from

Protein	11%
Fat	2%
Carbohydrate	87%

Tropical Smoothies

Try these exotic variations on the traditional fruit smoothie.

TIP

For a thinner consistency, add extra ice cubes.

Pineapple Banana

1 cup	chopped banana	250 mL
1 cup	pineapple juice	250 mL
½ cup to 1 cup	ice cubes	125 to 250 mL

1. In a blender, purée banana, pineapple juice and ice cubes. Pour into glasses and serve.

Pineapple Banana: **Nutritional value** Per Serving

Calories: 110, Protein: 1 g, Fat: 0 g, Carbohydrate: 27 g, Dietary Fiber: 1 g, Calcium: 25 mg
Percent of calories from Protein: 3%, Fat: 2%, Carbohydrate: 95%

Pineapple Coconut

1 cup	drained crushed pineapple	250 mL
1 cup	canned coconut milk	250 mL
½ cup to 1 cup	ice cubes	125 to 250 mL

1. In a blender, purée pineapple, coconut milk and ice cubes. Pour into glasses and serve.

Pineapple Coconut: **Nutritional value** Per Serving

Calories: 295, Protein: 3 g, Fat: 26 g, Carbohydrate: 19 g, Dietary Fiber: 1 g, Calcium: 38 mg
Percent of calories from Protein: 4%, Fat: 73%, Carbohydrate: 23%

Kiwi Passion Fruit

1 cup	chopped kiwi	250 mL
1 cup	passion fruit juice	250 mL
½ cup to 1 cup	ice cubes	125 to 250 mL

1. In a blender, purée kiwi, passion fruit juice and ice cubes. Pour into glasses and serve.

Kiwi Passion Fruit: **Nutritional value** Per Serving

Calories: 121, Protein: 2 g, Fat: 1 g, Carbohydrate: 31 g, Dietary Fiber: 3 g (a source), Calcium: 38 mg
Percent of calories from Protein: 5%, Fat: 4%, Carbohydrate: 92%

Banana Peanut Butter Smoothie

A classic combination, in drink form!

MAKES 1 SERVING

1	banana, chopped	1
1 cup	lactose-free milk or fortified soy milk	250 mL
2 tbsp	smooth peanut butter	25 mL

1. In a blender, purée banana, milk and peanut butter. Pour into a glass and serve.

Nutritional value
Per serving

Calories	398
Protein	17 g
Fat	20 g
Carbohydrate	45 g
Dietary Fiber (a high source)	4 g
Calcium (a very high source)	322 mg

Percent of calories from

Protein	16%
Fat	42%
Carbohydrate	42%

Cappuccino

You don't need a fancy coffee machine to make this popular beverage, specially designed for the lactose intolerant.

MAKES 1 SERVING

TIP

For best results, use a full-bodied coffee.

½ cup	lactose-free milk or fortified soy milk	125 mL
1 cup	hot filter espresso coffee	250 mL
	Unsweetened cocoa powder, ground cinnamon and granulated sugar	

1. In a small saucepan, heat milk over medium-high until steaming (or, in a microwave-safe bowl, microwave on High for 2 minutes). Whisk until frothy, then pour over coffee. Stir lightly. Sprinkle with cocoa, cinnamon and sugar as desired.

Nutritional value
Per serving

Calories	55
Protein	4 g
Fat	1 g
Carbohydrate	7 g
Dietary Fiber	0 g
Calcium (a source)	156 mg

Percent of calories from

Protein	31%
Fat	21%
Carbohydrate	49%

Café au Lait

Here's an excellent way to get a boost of calcium with your coffee.

MAKES 1 SERVING

TIP

To produce frothy milk, beat it with a whisk.

1 cup	hot strong coffee	250 mL
1 cup	lactose-free milk or fortified soy milk	250 mL
	Ground cinnamon and granulated sugar	

1. In a small saucepan, heat milk over medium-high until steaming (or, in a microwave-safe bowl, microwave on High for 2 minutes). Pour into coffee and stir. Sprinkle with cinnamon and sugar as desired.

Nutritional value
Per serving

Calories	106
Protein	8 g
Fat	3 g
Carbohydrate	13 g
Dietary Fiber	0 g
Calcium (a very high source)	308 mg

Percent of calories from

Protein	31%
Fat	22%
Carbohydrate	47%

Chocolate Milkshake

An old favorite, this version can be enjoyed by the lactose intolerant.

MAKES 1 SERVING

| 1 cup | fortified chocolate soy milk | 250 mL |
| ¼ cup | chocolate syrup | 50 mL |

1. Fill an ice cube tray with soy milk. Freeze for 1 to 2 hours, or until starting to firm.

2. In a blender, process partially frozen soy milk cubes and chocolate syrup until ice is finely chopped and drink is frothy. Pour into a glass and serve.

Nutritional value
Per serving

Calories	349
Protein	7 g
Fat	4 g
Carbohydrate	72 g
Dietary Fiber	0 g
Calcium (a very high source)	311 mg

Percent of calories from

Protein	8%
Fat	11%
Carbohydrate	82%

Celebration Menus

Typically, North American celebrations are full of rich food dressed in buttery sauces with a creamy dessert to finish. I hope these menu ideas will help those planning a lactose-free event to make it as much a celebration for lactose-intolerant people as it is for everyone else.

Adult Birthday Dinner

This menu is ideal for a simple yet tasty summer birthday barbecue. It is particularly appealing to men and teens, who enjoy these robust tastes.

> *Filet Mignon:* Instead of the usual garlic butter, rub the steak with a clove of garlic, grind fresh pepper over top and brush with extra-virgin olive oil before grilling. Serve with a horseradish sauce.
> *Caesar Salad with Creamy Garlic Dressing* (page 86)
> *Baked Potatoes* with *Tofu "Sour Cream"* (page 248)
> *Tomato Basil Salad* (page 93, see box)
> *Fudge Cake* (page 223) with *Vanilla Ice Cream* (page 236)

A Child's Birthday Party

Preparing a children's party can be an intimidating experience. Children let you know if they like something or not. Over the years, I have found that putting out a selection of foods for them to make their own works well. You control what is put out on trays, and they control what they eat. The only item that is fully prepared is the fruit punch, which always seems to be a hit.

> *Veggies and Dip:* Put out a selection of crudités. Make sure you include carrots, because they are usually the most popular. My choice for dip would be something relatively plain. Most kids love garlic: use the Creamy Garlic Dressing (page 86) or the basic Tofu Cream (page 247).
> *Make-Your-Own Pitas:* Put out a basket of pitas, cut in half for easy stuffing, along with bowls of shredded lettuce, grated carrot, sliced cucumber, pickles, sunflower sprouts, chopped egg, tuna salad and shredded smoked chicken.
> *Decorated Cupcakes:* Using the Basic Sponge Cake (page 220) or Fudge Cake (page 223) recipe, pour batter into colorful paper liners. Preheat oven to 350°F (180°C) and bake for 20 to 25 minutes, or until firm to the touch and a tester inserted in the center comes out clean. Put out trays of cupcakes with

bowls of Old-Fashioned Chocolate Sauce (page 261) or Lemon Butter (page 255) to dip cupcakes into. Set out bowls with sugar-based candies like jujubes or sprinkles for the kids to decorate their cakes. Do not include chocolate candies like Smarties® because they contain lactose.

Fruit Punch: Somehow, a fruit punch is always special. Cranberry-raspberry mixed with ginger ale and peach cocktail with ginger ale are two popular combinations, although lemonade always seems to work well too. Float some strawberries, sliced oranges, lemon or limes on top to make it look festive.

Thanksgiving

Herb-Roasted Turkey (page 144)

Loaf Pan Carrot Stuffing (page 167)

Creamy Sweet Potatoes: Cook sweet potatoes in water until tender and mash with a little fortified orange juice and brown sugar. An electric mixer works well to make them smooth and creamy. Season to taste with salt and pepper.

Green Beans with Almonds: Cook beans in boiling salted water. Drain. Toss with about 1 tbsp (15 mL) extra-virgin olive oil and a squeeze of lemon. Give this vegetable dish a calcium boost with a sprinkling of coarsely chopped toasted unblanched almonds (see tip, page 74). Just before serving, sprinkle over beans.

Pumpkin Pie (page 218) with *Vanilla Ice Cream* (page 236)

Festive Season

The festive season is always a hectic time of year, but this streamlined menu allows the chief cook time off to enjoy the day, since everything except the turkey can be done in advance. Even the turkey is a lazy cook's dream.

Salted Almonds (page 49)

Herb-Roasted Turkey (page 144)

Loaf Pan Carrot Stuffing (page 167)

Carrot Squash Crumble (page 168)

Mashed Potato Casserole (page 171)

Shortbread (page 214)

Yule Log (page 221, variation)

Spring

Baked Ham: Ham is lactose-free, providing the glaze chosen contains no milk products. A simple glaze of honey-mustard is delicious. Bake according to directions on the label.

Scalloped Potatoes (page 169)

Carrots with Maple Syrup (page 166)

Spring Salad with Oriental Flavors (page 84)

Lemon Torte made from **Basic Meringue** (page 215) spread with **Lemon Butter** (page 255)

Putting on the Ritz

Artichokes with Spicy Lemon Sauce (page 163)

Grilled Salmon (page 152)

Salad of Fresh Spring Greens, New Potatoes and Asparagus (page 92)

Jelly Roll made from **Basic Sponge Cake** (page 220) spread with **Lime Butter** (page 255, variation)

Nutrient Analysis

The nutrient analysis done on the recipes in this book is derived from The Food Processor SQL, version 9.7 (2005) Recipes are evaluated as follows:

- When there is a range of servings, the smaller of the two numbers and therefore the larger portion is selected.
- When optional ingredients are listed, they are not evaluated.
- When salt, pepper or confectioner's (icing) sugar is not quantified, it is not calculated in the analysis.
- When a choice is given for ingredients — for example, liquid honey or corn syrup — only the first is used in the calculation.
- Recipes listing variations are evaluated only for the basic or initial recipe.

The evaluation of recipe servings as sources of nutrients combine U.S. and Canadian regulations. Bearing in mind that the two countries have different reporting standards, the highest standard was always used As a result, some recipes that would have been identified as a very high source of a particular nutrient in one country may be listed only as a source or a high source because the standard is higher in the other country.

Note: Numbers for "percent of calories from" may not always total 100 due to rounding or because elements in addition to carbohydrate, protein and fat make up the total

Library and Archives Canada Cataloguing in Publication

Main, Jan
    200 best lactose-free recipes / Jan Main.

Includes index.
ISBN-13: 978-0-7788-0135-1
ISBN-10: 0-7788-0135-7

1. Milk-free diet—Recipes. I. Title. II. Title: Two hundred best lactose-free recipes.

RM234.5.M36 2006   641.5'6318   C2005-906118-9

Index

A

almonds
Amaretto Cheesecake, 225
Biscuit Tortoni, 235
Bread Pudding, 211
Caramelized Peach Rice
Gâteau, 222
Carrot, Apple and Almond
Muffins, 204
Carrot Squash Crumble, 168
Celebration Bread, 184
Chocolate Mousse, 234
Cocktail Crunch, 48
Cucumber Almond Salad, 96
Curried Parsnip Soup, 74
Drained Yogurt Cheesecake,
228
Dried Fruit Compote, 209
Dried Fruit with Goat
Cheese, 50
Fruited Truffles, 210
Green Beans with Almonds,
273
Layered Salad with Ranch-
Style Dressing, 88
Loaf Pan Carrot Stuffing, 167
Mushroom Strudel, 46
Nice 'n' Nutty Slaw, 102
Orange, Almond and Apricot
Tea Bread, 193
Orange Almond Scone, 198
Pasta with Calcium Greens
and Almonds, 106
Pear Ginger Cake, 195
Risotto, 173
Salted Almonds, 49
Sesame Crunch, 208
Spinach, Almond and
Orange Salad with Creamy
Tarragon Dressing, 94
Swedish Tea Ring, 181
Tuna Noodle Casserole, 116
Whole-Grain Seed and Nut
Bread, 186
Amaretto Cheesecake, 225
Amaretto Cream, 257
Antojitos, 38

apple
Apple Butter, 254
Apple French Toastwich, 55
Apple Jelly Roll or Sponge
Layer Cake, 221
Broccoli Apple Salad with
Creamy Curry Dressing,
90
Carrot, Apple and Almond
Muffins, 204
Cranberry Apple Muffins,
200
Creamy Pumpkin and Apple
Soup, 78
Creamy Stovetop Rice
Pudding, 212
Nice 'n' Nutty Slaw, 102
Pumpkin Butter, 252
Rossolye Salad, 98
Tofu Fruit Smoothie, 265
Yogurt Fruit Smoothie
(variation), 266
apricots, dried
Apricot Sorbet, 240
Creamy Chicken Curry,
138
Drained Yogurt Cheesecake,
228
Dried Fruit Compote, 209
Dried Fruit with Goat
Cheese, 50
Fruited Truffles, 210
Oatmeal Shortbread with
Date Filling (variation),
216
Orange, Almond and Apricot
Tea Bread, 193
Artichokes with Spicy Lemon
Sauce, 163
asparagus
Far East Noodles, 110
Salad of Fresh Spring
Greens, New Potatoes and
Asparagus, 92
Salmon and Wild Rice Salad
(tip), 100
Spring Salad with Oriental
Flavors, 84

B

bacon
Basic Quiche, 66
Creamy Clam Chowder, 82
Mushroom Chowder, 80
Baked Ham, 274
bananas
Banana Bran Muffins with
Cinnamon Sugar Topping,
203
Banana Citrus Loaf, 191
Banana Peanut Butter
Smoothie, 268
Banana Sorbet, 239
Basic Berry Smoothie, 264
Tofu Fruit Smoothie, 265
Tropical Coffee Cake, 194
Tropical Smoothies, 267
Yogurt Fruit Smoothie,
266
Basic Béchamel Sauce for
Chicken Dishes, 243
Basic Berry Smoothie, 264
Basic Chicken Stock, 68
Basic Cream Sauce, 242
Basic Crêpes, 62
Basic Custard, 207
Basic Custard Sauce, 262
Basic Meringue, 215
Basic Quiche, 66
Basic Sponge Cake, 220
Basic Yeast Bread, 177
beans. See also beans, green;
soybeans
Chicken Chili (variation),
133
Layered Salad with Ranch-
Style Dressing, 88
Minestrone, 72
New-Fashioned Bean Pot,
174
Pitas Stuffed with Hummus
and Sprouts, 39
Soybean Hummus, 28
Tex-Mex Bean and Salsa
Pyramid Dip, 25
Vegetarian Chili, 132

beans, green
Green Beans with Almonds, 273
Pasta Salad, 104
Salmon and Wild Rice Salad (tip), 100
Béchamel Sauce, 114, 118, 122
for Chicken Dishes, 243
Béchamel Tofu Sauce, 120
beef
Beef Stroganoff, 158
Burgers with the Works, 155
Florentine Lasagna, 122
Shepherd's Pie (variation), 140
Vegetarian Chili (variation), 132
Beer Bread, 187
Berry Smoothie, Basic, 264
beverages, 263–71
bioavailability, 16
birthday meals, 272–73
Biscuit Tortoni, 235
biscuits, 196–97
blueberries
Basic Berry Smoothie, 264
Blueberry Cornbread, 189
Quick Strawberry Sauce (variation), 259
Tofu Fruit Smoothie, 265
bok choy
Chicken Tofu Noodle Soup (variation), 70
Far East Noodles, 110
Fisherman's Pie (tip), 148
Frittata (variation), 64
Greek Salad (variation), 85
Nice 'n' Nutty Slaw (variation), 102
No-Fuss Mac and Cheese, 115
Stir-fry of Greens, 161
Tuna Noodle Casserole (variation), 116
Bow Knots, 178
Braided Loaf, 178
Braised Kale, 162

bran
Banana Bran Muffins with Cinnamon Sugar Topping, 203
Easy Health Bread, 182
Good Morning Bran Muffins, 201
Whole-Grain Seed and Nut Bread, 186
breads
quick, 175, 186–95, 197
yeast, 175, 177–85
breakfast and brunch dishes, 51–66
broccoli
Broccoli Apple Salad with Creamy Curry Dressing, 90
Broccoli Soufflé, 164
Broccoli Tarragon Soup, 71
Chicken Divan, 135
Far East Noodles, 110
Frittata, 64
Garden Lasagna, 120
Lazy Lasagna (variation), 118
No-Fuss Mac and Cheese, 115
Pasta Salad, 104
Pasta with Calcium Greens and Almonds, 106
Risotto, 173
Salmon and Wild Rice Salad, 100
Stir-fry of Greens, 161
Tuna Noodle Casserole (variation), 116
Bruschetta Pizza, 126
buns, 178, 179
Burgers with the Works, 155

C

cabbage
Frittata (variation), 64
Greek Salad (variation), 85
Nice 'n' Nutty Slaw, 102
No-Fuss Mac and Cheese, 115
Risotto, 173
Salad of Fresh Spring Greens, New Potatoes and Asparagus (tip), 92

Spinach, Almond and Orange Salad with Creamy Tarragon Dressing (variation), 94
Caesar Salad with Creamy Garlic Dressing, 86
Café au Lait, 270
calcium, 14–16, 19–22, 275
Cappuccino, 269
Cappuccino Cookies, 213
Cappuccino Sauce, 260
Caramelized Peach Rice Gâteau, 222
Caraway Currant Soda Bread, 190
carrots
Carrot, Apple and Almond Muffins, 204
Carrot Squash Crumble, 168
Carrots with Maple Syrup, 166
Chicken Pot Pie with Leeks and Mushrooms, 136
Cream of Carrot Soup, 79
Loaf Pan Carrot Stuffing, 167
Spring Salad with Oriental Flavors, 84
Celebration Bread, 184
celebration menus, 272–74
celery
Broccoli Apple Salad with Creamy Curry Dressing, 90
Layered Salad with Ranch-Style Dressing, 88
Nice 'n' Nutty Slaw, 102
Pasta Salad, 104
Stir-fry of Greens, 161
cheese, 20. *See also specific types of cheese (below)*
Broccoli Soufflé, 164
Dried Fruit with Goat Cheese, 50
Four Onion Pizza with Rosemary, 130
Greek Salad, 85
cheese, Cheddar
Basic Cream Sauce (variation), 242
Basic Quiche, 66

Broccoli Soufflé (variation), 164
Frittata, 64
Macaroni and Cheese, 114
Nachos with Beans, 36
cheese, Parmesan
Caesar Salad with Creamy Garlic Dressing, 86
Cheese Sauce, 242
Four Onion Pizza with Rosemary, 130
French Onion Soup, 75
Margherita Pizza, 124
Mediterranean Crostini, 40
Pesto Pasta, 109
Pesto Pizza, 125
Pesto Sauce, 244
Risotto, 173
cheesecakes, 224–29
chicken
Apple French Toastwich, 55
Basic Chicken Stock, 68
Burgers with the Works (variation), 155
Chicken Chili, 133
Chicken Divan, 135
Chicken Fingers, 147
Chicken Fingers with Creamy Dipping Sauce, 142
Chicken Pot Pie with Leeks and Mushrooms, 136
Chicken Tofu Noodle Soup, 70
Chicken without Bother, 134
Creamy Chicken Curry, 138
Far East Noodles, 110
French Toastwich, 54
Shepherd's Pie, 140
Vegetarian Chili (variation), 132
chickpeas
Chicken Chili (variation), 133
Minestrone (variation), 72
Soybean Hummus, 28
Vegetarian Chili, 132
chili, 132–33
Chocolate Cheesecake Squares, 227
Chocolate Cream Filling, 258

Chocolate Jelly Roll or Sponge Layer Cake, 221
Chocolate Milkshake, 271
Chocolate Mousse, 234
Chocolate Sauce, Old-Fashioned, 261
Christmas dishes, 273
Citrus Butter, 255
Citrus Jelly Roll or Sponge Layer Cake, 221
Clam Chowder, Creamy, 82
Cocktail Crunch, 48
cocoa powder, unsweetened
Cappuccino Cookies, 213
Cappuccino Sauce, 260
Chocolate Cheesecake Squares, 227
Chocolate Jelly Roll or Sponge Layer Cake, 221
Chocolate Mousse, 234
Fudge Cake, 223
Fudge Pudding, 232
Mocha Ice Cream, 237
Old-Fashioned Chocolate Sauce, 261
Tiramisu, 230
Vanilla Cream Filling (variation), 258
coconut milk
Creamy Chicken Curry, 138
Tropical Smoothies, 267
coffee
Café au Lait, 270
Cappuccino, 269
Cappuccino Cookies, 213
Cappuccino Sauce, 260
Chocolate Mousse, 234
Coffee Cream Filling, 258
Coffee Ice Cream, 237
Fudge Cake, 223
Fudge Pudding, 232
Good Morning Bran Muffins, 201
Mocha Ice Cream, 237
Old-Fashioned Chocolate Sauce, 261
Tiramisu, 230
Coquilles St. Jacques, 149
cornmeal
Blueberry Cornbread, 189
Double Cornbread, 188

cranberries
Cranberry Apple Muffins, 200
Tofu Fruit Smoothie, 265
Cream of Carrot Soup, 79
Cream Sauce, Basic, 242
Creamy Chicken Curry, 138
Creamy Clam Chowder, 82
Creamy Curry Dressing, 90
Creamy Dill Dressing, 98
Creamy Garlic Dressing, 86
Creamy Leek and Tomato Pasta, 108
Creamy Mashed Potatoes with Garlic, 170
Creamy Pumpkin and Apple Soup, 78
Creamy Stovetop Rice Pudding, 212
Creamy Sweet Potatoes, 273
Creamy Tarragon Dressing, 94
Creamy Veggie Dip, 24
Crêpes, Basic, 62
Crescent-Shaped Rolls, 179
Crostini, Mediterranean, 40
Cucumber Almond Salad, 96
currants
Caraway Currant Soda Bread, 190
Celebration Bread, 184
Creamy Stovetop Rice Pudding, 212
Currant Scones, 199
Double Pumpkin Muffins, 202
Fudge Pudding, 232
Swedish Tea Ring, 181
Curried Parsnip Soup, 74
Custard, Basic, 207
Custard Sauce, Basic, 262

D
dates
Drained Yogurt Cheesecake, 228
Dried Fruit Compote, 209
Dried Fruit with Goat Cheese, 50
Good Morning Bran Muffins, 201

dates (continued)
  Oatmeal Shortbread with
    Date Filling, 216
desserts, 205–40
Dill Mustard Sauce, 246
Dilled Salmon Soufflé, 60
dips, 24–29
Double Cornbread, 188
Double Pumpkin Muffins, 202
Double Salmon Spread, 30
Drained Yogurt Cheesecake, 228
dressings, salad, 84–104
Dried Fruit Compote, 209
Dried Fruit with Goat Cheese,
  50

E

Easter dishes, 274
Easy Health Bread, 182
Easy Salmon Pie, 150
eggs
  Basic Custard, 207
  Basic Meringue, 215
  Basic Quiche, 66
  Broccoli Soufflé, 164
  Chocolate Mousse, 234
  Dilled Salmon Soufflé, 60
  Easy Salmon Pie, 150
  Frittata, 64
  Lemon Butter, 255
  Make-Ahead Scramble, 56
  Orange French Toast, 52
  Salmon Loaf, 154
  Tiramisu, 230
  Vanilla Ice Cream, 236

F

Far East Noodles, 110
Fettuccini Alfredo, 113
fiber, dietary, 275
figs, dried
  Drained Yogurt Cheesecake,
    228
  Dried Fruit Compote, 209
  Dried Fruit with Goat
    Cheese, 50
  Fruited Truffles, 210
  Oatmeal Shortbread with
    Date Filling (variation),
    216
Filet Mignon, 272

fish. See also specific types of fish;
    seafood
  Fish Fingers, 146
  Fisherman's Pie, 148
Florentine Lasagna, 122
Four Onion Pizza with
    Rosemary, 130
French Onion Soup, 75
French Potato Salad, 97
French toast, 52–55
French Toastwich, 54
Frittata, 64
frozen desserts, 236–40
fruit. See also specific fruits; fruit
    juices
  Basic Berry Smoothie, 264
  Biscuit Tortoni, 235
  Dried Fruit Compote, 209
  Dried Fruit with Goat
    Cheese, 50
  Fruited Truffles, 210
  Tropical Coffee Cake, 194
  Tropical Smoothies, 267
  Yogurt Fruit Smoothie, 266
fruit juices, 20. See also orange
    juice
  Apple Butter, 254
  Apple Jelly Roll or Sponge
    Layer Cake, 221
  Caramelized Peach Rice
    Gâteau, 222
  Creamy Stovetop Rice
    Pudding, 212
  Fruit Punch, 273
  Pumpkin Butter, 252
  Tofu Fruit Smoothie, 265
  Tropical Smoothies, 267
  Yogurt Fruit Smoothie, 266
Fudge Cake, 223
Fudge Pudding, 232

G

Garden Lasagna, 120
garlic
  Artichokes with Spicy
    Lemon Sauce, 163
  Bruschetta Pizza, 126
  Creamy Chicken Curry, 138
  Creamy Garlic Dressing, 86
  Four Onion Pizza with
    Rosemary, 130

  Garden Lasagna, 120
  Herbed Spiral Loaf, 180
  Pesto Sauce, 244
  Roasted Ratatouille Pizza,
    128
  Salsa, 34
  Shepherd's Pie, 140
  Vegetarian Chili, 132
Glazed Lemon Loaf, 192
Good Morning Bran Muffins,
  201
Greek Salad, 85
Green Beans with Almonds,
  273
Green Sauce, 245
Gremolata Bread Crumbs, 249
Grilled Salmon, 152
Guacamole Spread, 29

H

ham
  Apple French Toastwich, 55
  Baked Ham, 274
  French Toastwich, 54
  Linguine with Creamy
    Mushroom and Ham
    Sauce, 112
Hamburger Buns, 179
Health Bread, Easy, 182
Herb-Roasted Turkey, 144
Herbed Pâté, 33
Herbed Spiral Loaf, 180

J

jalapeño peppers. See peppers,
    jalapeño
Jelly Roll, 220

K

kale
  Braised Kale, 162
  Broccoli Soufflé (variation),
    164
  Chicken Tofu Noodle Soup
    (variation), 70
  Frittata (variation), 64
  Greek Salad (variation), 85
  Kale Tart with Sun-Dried
    Tomatoes and Pine Nuts,
    44
  Lazy Lasagna (variation), 118

Minestrone, 72
No-Fuss Mac and Cheese, 115
Pasta with Calcium Greens and Almonds, 106
Risotto, 173
Salad of Fresh Spring Greens, New Potatoes and Asparagus (tip), 92
Spinach, Almond and Orange Salad with Creamy Tarragon Dressing (variation), 94
Tuna Noodle Casserole (variation), 116

L

lactase tablets, 20
lactose intolerance, 11–13
lasagna, 118–23
Layered Salad with Ranch-Style Dressing, 88
Lazy Lasagna, 118
leeks
  Chicken Pot Pie with Leeks and Mushrooms, 136
  Chicken Tofu Noodle Soup, 70
  Creamy Clam Chowder, 82
  Creamy Leek and Tomato Pasta, 108
  Fisherman's Pie, 148
  Four Onion Pizza with Rosemary, 130
  Garden Lasagna, 120
  Leek and Potato Soup, 76
  Mushroom Strudel, 46
  Risotto, 173
lemon
  Amaretto Cheesecake, 225
  Amaretto Cream, 257
  Apricot Sorbet, 240
  Banana Citrus Loaf, 191
  Banana Sorbet, 239
  Basic Custard Sauce (variation), 262
  Basic Sponge Cake (variation), 220
  Blueberry Cornbread, 189
  Caramelized Peach Rice Gâteau, 222

Celebration Bread, 184
Cucumber Almond Salad, 96
Drained Yogurt Cheesecake, 228
Dried Fruit Compote, 209
Glazed Lemon Loaf, 192
Gremolata Bread Crumbs, 249
Lemon Butter, 255
Lemon Cheesecake, 224
Lemon Ice Cream, 237
Lemon Sesame Twists, 197
Pear Butter, 253
Pear Ginger Cake, 195
Risotto, 173
Salmon-Stuffed Baked Potatoes, 172
lettuce
  Caesar Salad with Creamy Garlic Dressing, 86
  Greek Salad (variation), 85
  Nachos with Beans, 36
  Tex-Mex Bean and Salsa Pyramid Dip, 25
lime
  Lime Butter, 255
  Mango Sorbet, 238
  Mexican Tortilla Rolls, 37
Linguine with Creamy Mushroom and Ham Sauce, 112
liqueur
  Amaretto Cheesecake, 225
  Amaretto Cream, 257
  Biscuit Tortoni, 235
  Chocolate Mousse, 234
  Orange French Toast, 52
  Yogurt Sauce, 256
Loaf Pan Carrot Stuffing, 167
lunch dishes, 51–66

M

Macaroni and Cheese, 114
Make-Ahead Scramble, 56
Mango Sorbet, 238
Margherita Pizza, 124
marinades, 97
Marinated Tofu, 126
Mashed Potato Casserole, 171
meat dishes, 155–58
Mediterranean Crostini, 40

Meringue, Basic, 215
Mexican Tortilla Rolls, 37
milk, 14
  allergy to, 12, 13
  lactose-free, 20
  soy, 18–19, 20
Minestrone, 72
Mocha Cream Filling, 258
Mocha Ice Cream, 237
molasses
  Easy Health Bread, 182
  Good Morning Bran Muffins, 201
  Pumpkin Butter, 252
muffins, 188, 200–4
mushrooms
  Beef Stroganoff, 158
  Chicken Pot Pie with Leeks and Mushrooms, 136
  Far East Noodles, 110
  Fisherman's Pie, 148
  Florentine Lasagna, 122
  Garden Lasagna, 120
  Layered Salad with Ranch-Style Dressing, 88
  Linguine with Creamy Mushroom and Ham Sauce, 112
  Make-Ahead Scramble, 56
  Mushroom Chowder, 80
  Mushroom Cream Sauce, 243
  Mushroom Strudel, 46
  Pasta with Calcium Greens and Almonds, 106
  Roasted Ratatouille Pizza, 128
  Salmon and Wild Rice Salad, 100
  Shepherd's Pie, 140
  Stir-fry of Greens, 161
  Tuna Primavera, 145
  Veal and Mushrooms, 156

N

Nachos with Beans, 36
New-Fashioned Bean Pot, 174
Nice 'n' Nutty Slaw, 102
No-Fuss Mac and Cheese, 115

noodles. *See also* pasta
  Chicken Tofu Noodle Soup, 70
  Far East Noodles, 110
  Tuna Noodle Casserole, 116
nutrients, 275
nuts. *See also* almonds; pine nuts
  Creamy Chicken Curry, 138
  Whole-Grain Seed and Nut Bread, 186

O

oats, rolled (quick-cooking)
  Easy Health Bread, 182
  Oatmeal Shortbread with Date Filling, 216
  Sesame Crunch, 208
  Whole-Grain Seed and Nut Bread, 186
Old-Fashioned Chocolate Sauce, 261
olives
  Antojitos, 38
  Greek Salad, 85
  Herbed Pâté, 33
  Mexican Tortilla Rolls, 37
  Pasta Salad, 104
  Tex-Mex Bean and Salsa Pyramid Dip, 25
onions. *See also* onions, green
  Four Onion Pizza with Rosemary, 130
  French Onion Soup, 75
  Greek Salad, 85
  Layered Salad with Ranch-Style Dressing, 88
  Potato Tortilla, 58
  Roasted Ratatouille Pizza, 128
  Spinach, Almond and Orange Salad with Creamy Tarragon Dressing, 94
onions, green
  Creamy Veggie Dip, 24
  Far East Noodles, 110
  Herbed Spiral Loaf, 180
  Make-Ahead Scramble, 56
  Nice 'n' Nutty Slaw, 102
  Pasta Salad, 104

Pitas Stuffed with Hummus and Sprouts, 39
Salmon and Wild Rice Salad, 100
Tex-Mex Bean and Salsa Pyramid Dip, 25
Tuna Noodle Casserole, 116
orange. *See also* orange juice
  Banana Citrus Loaf, 191
  Basic Custard Sauce (variation), 262
  Blueberry Cornbread, 189
  Cranberry Apple Muffins, 200
  Fruited Truffles, 210
  Good Morning Bran Muffins, 201
  Lemon Butter (variation), 255
  Oatmeal Shortbread with Date Filling, 216
  Orange, Almond and Apricot Tea Bread, 193
  Orange Almond Scone, 198
  Orange French Toast, 52
  Orange Marmalade Sauce, 52
  Spinach, Almond and Orange Salad with Creamy Tarragon Dressing, 94
  Tropical Coffee Cake, 194
  Yogurt Fruit Smoothie, 266
orange juice
  Basic Berry Smoothie, 264
  Basic Custard, 207
  Basic Sponge Cake (variation), 220
  Carrot Squash Crumble, 168
  Chocolate Mousse, 234
  Creamy Stovetop Rice Pudding (variation), 212
  Creamy Sweet Potatoes, 273
  Dried Fruit Compote, 209
  Loaf Pan Carrot Stuffing, 167
  Orange Pancakes, 61
  Sweet Potato–Orange Soup, 77
  Tofu Fruit Smoothie, 265
Oriental Dressing, 84
osteoporosis, 15
oxalates, 16

P

Pan Buns, 178
pancakes, 61–63
Parsley Pesto, 27
Parsnip Soup, Curried, 74
pasta. *See also* noodles
  Chicken Tofu Noodle Soup, 70
  Creamy Leek and Tomato Pasta, 108
  Fettuccini Alfredo, 113
  Florentine Lasagna, 122
  Garden Lasagna, 120
  Lazy Lasagna, 118
  Linguine with Creamy Mushroom and Ham Sauce, 112
  Macaroni and Cheese, 114
  Pasta Salad, 104
  Pasta with Calcium Greens and Almonds, 106
  Pesto Pasta, 109
pâtés, 31–33
pears
  Curried Parsnip Soup, 74
  Pear Butter, 253
  Pear Ginger Cake, 195
peppers, bell
  Frittata, 64
  Layered Salad with Ranch-Style Dressing, 88
  Mexican Tortilla Rolls, 37
  New-Fashioned Bean Pot, 174
  Pasta Salad, 104
  Pasta with Calcium Greens and Almonds, 106
  Roasted Ratatouille Pizza, 128
  Salsa, 34
  Spring Salad with Oriental Flavors, 84
  Stir-fry of Greens, 161
  Tex-Mex Bean and Salsa Pyramid Dip, 25
  Vegetarian Chili, 132
peppers, jalapeño
  Antojitos, 38
  Salsa, 34
  Tofu "Sour Cream" for Baked Potatoes, 248

Pesto Pasta, 109
Pesto Pizza, 125
Pesto Sauce, 244
phyllo (strudel) dough
    Mushroom Strudel, 46
    Spanakopita, 42
phytates, 16
pine nuts
    Kale Tart with Sun-Dried
        Tomatoes and Pine Nuts, 44
    Pesto Sauce, 244
    Sun-Dried Tomato and
        Parsley Pesto Dip, 26
Pitas Stuffed with Hummus
    and Sprouts, 39
pizza, 124–30
poppy seeds
    Easy Health Bread, 182
    Poppy Seed Dressing, 102
    Tortilla Chips, 35
pork
    Far East Noodles, 110
    Veal and Mushrooms
        (variation), 156
potatoes. See also sweet
    potatoes
    Broccoli Tarragon Soup, 71
    Creamy Clam Chowder, 82
    Creamy Mashed Potatoes
        with Garlic, 170
    Fisherman's Pie, 148
    French Potato Salad, 97
    Leek and Potato Soup, 76
    Mashed Potato Casserole,
        171
    Mushroom Chowder, 80
    Potato Tortilla, 58
    Rossolye Salad, 98
    Salad of Fresh Spring
        Greens, New Potatoes and
        Asparagus, 92
    Salmon Chowder, 81
    Salmon-Stuffed Baked
        Potatoes, 172
    Scalloped Potatoes, 169
    Shepherd's Pie (variation),
        140
poultry dishes, 133–44
pumpkin purée
    Creamy Pumpkin and Apple
        Soup, 78

Double Pumpkin Muffins,
    202
Pumpkin Butter, 252
Pumpkin Pie, 218
pumpkin seeds
    Double Pumpkin Muffins,
        202
    Easy Health Bread, 182

Q

Quiche, Basic, 66
Quick Sauté of Collard Greens,
    160
Quick Strawberry Sauce, 259

R

raisins
    Bread Pudding, 211
    Celebration Bread, 184
    Creamy Stovetop Rice
        Pudding, 212
    Swedish Tea Ring, 181
Ranch-Style Dressing, 88
Raspberry Cheesecake in a
    Glass, 226
rice
    Caramelized Peach Rice
        Gâteau, 222
    Creamy Stovetop Rice
        Pudding, 212
    Easy Salmon Pie, 150
    Risotto, 173
    Salmon and Wild Rice Salad,
        100
Roasted Ratatouille Pizza,
    128
rolls, 178–79
Rosemary Sun-Dried Tomato
    Crumb Topping, 250
Rossolye Salad, 98
rum
    Fudge Pudding, 232
    Pumpkin Pie, 218
    Tiramisu, 230
    Yogurt Sauce, 256

S

salad dressings, 84–104
Salad of Fresh Spring Greens,
    New Potatoes and
    Asparagus, 92

salads, 83–103
salmon
    Basic Quiche (variation),
        66
    Dilled Salmon Soufflé, 60
    Double Salmon Spread, 30
    Easy Salmon Pie, 150
    Grilled Salmon, 152
    Salad of Fresh Spring
        Greens, New Potatoes and
        Asparagus (tip), 92
    Salmon and Wild Rice Salad,
        100
    Salmon Chowder, 81
    Salmon Loaf, 154
    Salmon Mousse, 153
    Salmon-Stuffed Baked
        Potatoes, 172
    Seafood Pâté, 32
    Smoked Salmon Pâté, 31
    Tuna Noodle Casserole
        (variation), 116
    Tuna Primavera (variation),
        145
Salsa, 34
salsa (as ingredient)
    Antojitos, 38
    Mexican Tortilla Rolls, 37
    Nachos with Beans, 36
    New-Fashioned Bean Pot,
        174
    No-Fuss Mac and Cheese,
        115
    Tex-Mex Bean and Salsa
        Pyramid Dip, 25
Salted Almonds, 49
sardines
    Caesar Salad with Creamy
        Garlic Dressing, 86
    Mediterranean Crostini, 40
    Rossolye Salad, 98
sauces
    savory, 41, 56, 114, 163,
        242–46
    sweet, 52, 256–57, 259–62
Savory Sesame Biscuits, 196
Scalloped Potatoes, 169
scones, 198–99
seafood
    Coquilles St. Jacques, 149
    Seafood Pâté, 32

sesame seeds
 Broccoli Apple Salad with Creamy Curry Dressing, 90
 Chicken Fingers with Creamy Dipping Sauce, 142
 Cocktail Crunch, 48
 Double Pumpkin Muffins, 202
 Easy Health Bread, 182
 Far East Noodles, 110
 Nice 'n' Nutty Slaw, 102
 Sesame Crunch, 208
 Sesame Tea Biscuits, 196
 Spring Salad with Oriental Flavors, 84
 Stir-fry of Greens, 161
 Tortilla Chips, 35
 Whole-Grain Seed and Nut Bread, 186
shallots
 Fettuccini Alfredo, 113
 Four Onion Pizza with Rosemary, 130
Shepherd's Pie, 140
sherry
 Basic Béchamel Sauce for Chicken Dishes, 243
 Beef Stroganoff, 158
 Linguine with Creamy Mushroom and Ham Sauce, 112
Shortbread, 214
Smoked Salmon Pâté, 31
smoothies, 264–68
soups, 67–82
sour cream substitutes, 71, 248
soybean products, 16–19
 soy milk, 18–19, 20
soybeans
 Chicken Chili, 133
 Lazy Lasagna (variation), 118
 Minestrone, 72
 Pasta Salad, 104
 Soybean Hummus, 28
 Vegetarian Chili, 132
Spanakopita, 42
Spicy Lemon Sauce, 163

spinach
 Garden Lasagna, 120
 Layered Salad with Ranch-Style Dressing, 88
 Spanakopita, 42
 Spinach, Almond and Orange Salad with Creamy Tarragon Dressing, 94
Sponge Cake, Basic, 220
spreads
 savory, 29–33
 sweet, 252–55
Spring Salad with Oriental Flavors, 84
sprouts, sunflower or alfalfa
 Broccoli Apple Salad with Creamy Curry Dressing, 90
 Nice 'n' Nutty Slaw, 102
 Pitas Stuffed with Hummus and Sprouts, 39
 Tex-Mex Bean and Salsa Pyramid Dip, 25
squash
 Carrot Squash Crumble, 168
 Cream of Carrot Soup (variation), 79
 Roasted Ratatouille Pizza (variation), 128
Stir-fry of Greens, 161
strawberries
 Basic Berry Smoothie, 264
 Quick Strawberry Sauce, 259
 Strawberry Ice Cream, 237
 Tofu Fruit Smoothie, 265
strudel (phyllo) dough
 Mushroom Strudel, 46
 Spanakopita, 42
stuffing, 167
Sun-Dried Tomato and Parsley Pesto Dip, 26
Swedish Tea Ring, 181
sweet potatoes
 Creamy Mashed Potatoes with Garlic (variation), 170
 Shepherd's Pie, 140
 Sweet Potato–Orange Soup, 77

T
Tarragon Dressing, Creamy, 94
Tex-Mex Bean and Salsa Pyramid Dip, 25
Thanksgiving dishes, 273
Tiramisu, 230
tofu, 10, 16–17, 18–19. See also tofu, firm; tofu, soft
tofu, firm
 Amaretto Cheesecake, 225
 Bruschetta Pizza, 126
 Chicken Tofu Noodle Soup, 70
 Far East Noodles, 110
 Kale Tart with Sun-Dried Tomatoes and Pine Nuts, 44
 Lazy Lasagna (variation), 118
 Lemon Cheesecake, 224
 Mexican Tortilla Rolls, 37
 Mushroom Strudel, 46
 Spanakopita, 42
 Spring Salad with Oriental Flavors, 84
 Tofu "Sour Cream" for Baked Potatoes, 248
tofu, soft
 Amaretto Cream, 257
 Antojitos, 38
 Broccoli Apple Salad with Creamy Curry Dressing, 90
 Caesar Salad with Creamy Garlic Dressing, 86
 Chocolate Cheesecake Squares, 227
 Double Salmon Spread, 30
 Garden Lasagna, 120
 Green Sauce, 245
 Guacamole Spread, 29
 Herbed Pâté, 33
 Kale Tart with Sun-Dried Tomatoes and Pine Nuts, 44
 Layered Salad with Ranch-Style Dressing, 88
 Make-Ahead Scramble, 56
 Raspberry Cheesecake in a Glass, 226
 Rossolye Salad, 98

Salmon Mousse, 153
Seafood Pâté, 32
Smoked Salmon Pâté, 31
Sour Cream Substitute, 71
Spinach, Almond and
    Orange Salad with Creamy
    Tarragon Dressing, 94
Sun-Dried Tomato and
    Parsley Pesto Dip, 26
Tex-Mex Bean and Salsa
    Pyramid Dip, 25
Tiramisu, 230
Tofu Cream, 247
Tofu Fruit Smoothie, 265
Yogurt Substitute, 71
tomato. See also tomato,
    sun-dried
Beef Stroganoff, 158
Bruschetta Pizza, 126
Chicken Chili, 133
Creamy Leek and Tomato
    Pasta, 108
Florentine Lasagna, 122
Greek Salad, 85
Lazy Lasagna, 118
Margherita Pizza, 124
Mediterranean Crostini, 40
Minestrone, 72
Pesto Pizza, 125
Salad of Fresh Spring
    Greens, New Potatoes and
    Asparagus, 92
Salsa, 34
Tomato Basil Salad, 93
Tomato Sauce, Homemade, 41
Vegetarian Chili, 132
tomato, sun-dried
Caesar Salad with Creamy
    Garlic Dressing, 86
Kale Tart with Sun-Dried
    Tomatoes and Pine Nuts,
    44
Rosemary Sun-Dried Tomato
    Crumb Topping, 250
Sesame Tea Biscuits
    (variation), 196
Sun-Dried Tomato and
    Parsley Pesto Dip, 26
toppings
bread crumb, 58, 114, 121,
    123, 135

savory, 168, 247–51
sweet, 258
tortillas (as ingredient)
Antojitos, 38
Mexican Tortilla Rolls, 37
Tortilla Chips, 35
Tropical Coffee Cake, 194
Tropical Smoothies, 267
tuna
Tuna Noodle Casserole,
    116
Tuna Primavera, 145
turkey
Apple French Toastwich, 55
Basic Chicken Stock
    (variation), 68
Burgers with the Works
    (variation), 155
Chicken Tofu Noodle Soup
    (variation), 70
French Toastwich, 54
Herb-Roasted Turkey, 144
Linguine with Creamy
    Mushroom and Ham
    Sauce, 112
Shepherd's Pie, 140
Turkey Sausages, 143
Turkey Stock, 69

V

Vanilla Cream Filling, 258
Vanilla Ice Cream, 236
Veal and Mushrooms, 156
vegetables, 159–74. See also
    specific vegetables
Creamy Veggie Dip, 24
Double Cornbread, 188
Garden Lasagna, 120
Greek Salad, 85
Guacamole Spread, 29
Nice 'n' Nutty Slaw, 102
Parsley Pesto, 27
Pesto Sauce, 244
Quick Sauté of Collard
    Greens, 160
Roasted Ratatouille Pizza,
    128
Rossolye Salad, 98
Salad of Fresh Spring
    Greens, New Potatoes and
    Asparagus, 92

Salmon and Wild Rice Salad,
    100
Spring Salad with Oriental
    Flavors, 84
Sun-Dried Tomato and
    Parsley Pesto Dip, 26
Vegetarian Chili, 132
vitamin D, 14, 19, 20

W

Whole-Grain Seed and Nut
    Bread, 186
Whole Wheat Bread, 177
Whole Wheat Croutons, 251
wine (white)
Basic Béchamel Sauce for
    Chicken Dishes, 243
Chicken without Bother,
    134
Fisherman's Pie, 148
Linguine with Creamy
    Mushroom and Ham
    Sauce, 112
Mushroom Chowder, 80
Risotto, 173
Salmon Chowder, 81

Y

Yeast Blini, 63
Yeast Bread, Basic, 177
yogurt, 20
Broccoli Tarragon Soup, 71
Creamy Chicken Curry, 138
Currant Scones, 199
Drained Yogurt Cheesecake,
    228
Lemon Sesame Twists, 197
Sesame Tea Biscuits, 196
Yogurt Fruit Smoothie, 266
Yogurt Sauce, 256
yogurt substitute, 71
Yule Log, 221

Z

zucchini
Roasted Ratatouille Pizza,
    128
Salmon and Wild Rice Salad
    (variation), 100

More Great Books from Robert Rose

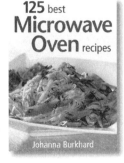

Appliance Cooking

- 125 Best Microwave Oven Recipes
  by Johanna Burkhard
- The Blender Bible
  by Andrew Chase and Nicole Young
- The Mixer Bible
  by Meredith Deeds and Carla Snyder
- The 150 Best Slow Cooker Recipes
  by Judith Finlayson
- Delicious & Dependable Slow Cooker Recipes
  by Judith Finlayson
- 125 Best Vegetarian Slow Cooker Recipes
  by Judith Finlayson
- 125 Best Rotisserie Oven Recipes
  by Judith Finlayson
- 125 Best Food Processor Recipes
  by George Geary
- The Best Family Slow Cooker Recipes
  by Donna-Marie Pye
- The Best Convection Oven Cookbook
  by Linda Stephen
- 125 Best Toaster Oven Recipes
  by Linda Stephen
- 250 Best American Bread Machine Baking Recipes
  by Donna Washburn and Heather Butt
- 250 Best Canadian Bread Machine Baking Recipes
  by Donna Washburn and Heather Butt

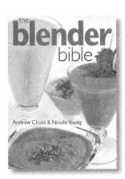

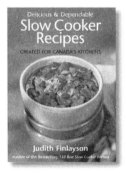

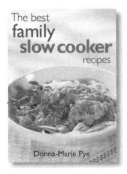

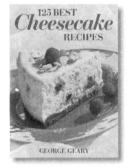

Baking

- 250 Best Cakes & Pies
  by Esther Brody
- 500 Best Cookies, Bars & Squares
  by Esther Brody
- 500 Best Muffin Recipes
  by Esther Brody
- 125 Best Cheesecake Recipes
  by George Geary
- 125 Best Chocolate Recipes
  by Julie Hasson
- 125 Best Chocolate Chip Recipes
  by Julie Hasson
- 125 Best Cupcake Recipes
  by Julie Hasson
- Complete Cake Mix Magic
  by Jill Snider

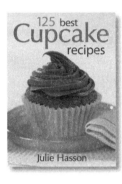

Healthy Cooking

- 125 Best Vegetarian Recipes
  by Byron Ayanoglu with contributions from Algis Kemezys
- America's Best Cookbook for Kids with Diabetes
  by Colleen Bartley
- Canada's Best Cookbook for Kids with Diabetes
  by Colleen Bartley
- The Juicing Bible
  by Pat Crocker and Susan Eagles
- The Smoothies Bible
  by Pat Crocker

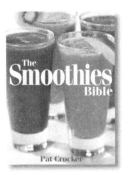

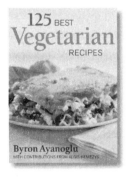